Safe and Healthy Schools

The Guilford Practical Intervention in the Schools Series

Kenneth W. Merrell, Series Editor

Safe and Healthy Schools

Practical Prevention Strategies

JEFFREY R. SPRAGUE
HILL M. WALKER

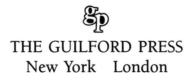

THE GUILFORD PRESS
New York   London

© 2005 The Guilford Press
A Division of Guilford Publications, Inc.
72 Spring Street, New York, NY 10012
www.guilford.com

Printed in Canada

This book is printed on acid-free paper.

Last digit is print number: 9 8 7 6 5 4 3 2 1

Library of Congress Cataloging-in-Publication Data

Sprague, Jeffrey R. (Jeffrey Richard), 1956–
   Safe and healthy schools : practical prevention strategies / Jeffrey R. Sprague, Hill M. Walker.
       p. cm.—(Guilford practical intervention in the schools series)
   Includes bibliographical references and index.
   ISBN 1-59385-105-7 (pbk. : alk. paper)
   1. Schools—United States—Safety measures. 2. School violence—United States—Prevention. I. Walker, Hill M. II. Title. III. Series.
   LB2866.S67 2005
   371.7′82—dc22
                                                                                            2004021183

About the Authors

Jeffrey R. Sprague PhD, is Associate Professor of Special Education and Codirector of the Institute on Violence and Destructive Behavior at the University of Oregon. In 2001, Dr. Sprague worked with the Oregon legislature to establish the Oregon Center for School Safety. Previously a classroom teacher and a school behavioral consultant, Dr. Sprague was also the Director of the Center for School and Community Integration at the Indiana University Institute for the Study of Developmental Disabilities. He has directed federal, state, and local research and demonstration projects related to whole-school discipline, youth violence prevention, alternative education, juvenile delinquency prevention, school inclusion, school-to-work transition and employment, school systems change, and self-advocacy. His research activities encompass applied behavior analysis, positive behavior supports, functional behavioral assessment, school safety and violence prevention, and juvenile delinquency. A contributor to "Early Warning, Timely Response," and the "President's Annual Reports on School Safety" in 1998, 1999, and 2000, Dr. Sprague has recently written a white paper on school safety for Oregon Attorney General Hardy Myers's School Safety Coalition and the book *Safe School Design: A Handbook for Educational Leaders Applying the Principles of Crime Prevention through Environmental Design* (with Tod Schneider and Hill M. Walker).

Hill M. Walker, PhD, is Professor of Special Education, Codirector of the Institute on Violence and Destructive Behavior, and Director of the Center on Human Development in the College of Education at the University of Oregon. He has a longstanding interest in behavioral assessment and in the development of effective intervention procedures with a range of behavior disorders for use in school settings. He has been engaged in applied research throughout his career, and his research interests include social skills assessment, curriculum development and intervention, longitudinal studies of aggression and antisocial behavior, and the development of early screening procedures for detecting students who are at risk for social–behavioral adjustment problems and/or later school dropout. Dr. Walker's most recent books include *Interventions for Academic and Behavior Problems II: Preventive and Remedial Approaches* (coedited with Mark Shinn and Gary Stoner) and the second edition of *Antisocial Behavior in School: Evidence-Based Practices* (coauthored with Elizabeth Ramsey and Frank M. Gresham).

Preface

In the 1990s, our public schools and nation were profoundly shaken by a series of school shootings that changed the landscape of school safety and forever altered the sense of safety and predictability that students, parents, and educators have traditionally held about the schooling process and the school building itself. In the wake of these tragedies, students and parents were traumatized on a broad scale by fears of school shootings and concerns about lack of school security. Even though our schools, compared to the community at large, are one of the safest places for our children and youth, they are no longer regarded as safe havens in which students are free to develop academically and socially without concern for their physical and emotional safety.

In the rush to understand the causes of these tragedies, and to find solutions, multiple and disparate research and practice traditions have begun to merge into a relatively distinct field of school safety research. Contributing disciplines to this field include public health, criminology, psychology, special education, prevention science, security, and many others. There is now a research journal (the *Journal of School Violence*) that focuses on school safety, and entire conferences are dedicated to the subject. However, while careful research can help to determine the most likely causes for school violence and provide effective solutions, its application needs to be monitored closely to avoid the risk of overwhelming school and community leaders with complicated, or even conflicting, information.

Practice generally lags well behind the research that validates evidence-based approaches, which inform and guide the policies and procedures on which they are based. This is especially true in the area of school safety and violence prevention. The pressures and demands of the moment force school and community leaders into making decisions about school safety strategies and tactics that may appear promising but may not be as yet proven through the research process. Thus, these leaders are left to base their decisions, for the most part, on their experience and best judgment. Until the knowledge base on school safety becomes more solid and cohesive, evidence-based practices will most likely not be consistently adopted or used.

HOW THIS BOOK CAN HELP YOU MAKE YOUR SCHOOL SAFER

This book is designed to assist school personnel and others to assess, select, and implement evidence-based school safety and prevention practices. The content and recommendations are based on our experience assisting hundreds of schools across the United States (including seven of the federally funded Safe Schools/Healthy Students communities), our careful review of the literature on school safety and antisocial behavior, and our own original research into the area. The book's chapters are briefly described below:

Chapter 1. At-Risk Youth and School Safety. This chapter provides a comprehensive overview of the challenges and context of school safety and sets the stage for the remainder of the book.

Chapter 2. Developing a Comprehensive School Safety and Prevention Plan. This chapter outlines a strategy, moving from needs assessment to intervention selection to program evaluation. Recommended assessment tools and a decision framework for intervention selection are presented.

Chapter 3. Improving School Climate, Safety, and Student Health with Schoolwide Positive Behavior Supports. We describe a system for implementing positive behavior support methods at the schoolwide level. Schoolwide positive behavior supports provide an integrated, sustainable system of supports for students and school professionals, and are the foundation for all school safety approaches.

Chapter 4. Bullying and Peer-Based Harassment in Schools. This chapter reviews the general characteristics, dynamics, and prevalence of the bully/victim problem in today's schools. It discusses some legal and policy implications, as well as system-based solutions to this increasing problem, intended for use by school personnel.

Chapter 5. Solutions for Bullying and Peer Harassment in the School Setting. The material in this chapter outlines strategies for preventing, ameliorating, and remediating the growing problem of bullying and peer harassment in our schools. Some considerations for school personnel responsible for addressing bullying and harassment are provided next, prior to the description of recommended intervention strategies.

Chapter 6. Screening and Identifying Behaviorally At-Risk Students. This chapter frames the critical issues and characterizes the landscape around early risk factors and the warning signs of potential violence. We describe recommended screening approaches in this area for use by school personnel. Access to this knowledge base is essential for every adult working in today's schools.

Chapter 7. Supporting Antisocial and Potentially Violent Youth. Students who engage in antisocial and potentially violent behavior in school and other settings have complex and diverse support needs. These students often lead lives characterized by circumstances known to predict life-course juvenile delinquency, such as poverty, poor parental supervision, living in crime-ridden neighborhoods, and associating with delinquent peers. Given these circumstances, it is easy to understand why many behaviorally at-risk students experience serious adjustment problems that demand significant administrative time, disrupt regular classroom instruction, fail to respond to traditional school discipline, and, in some cases, pose a serious threat to the safety of other students or school staff. When not in school, these youth lack supervision and affiliate with other at-risk peers—circumstances that can easily lead to their involvement in juvenile crime. This chapter outlines a recommended approach for schools that is feasible and based on the best intervention research.

It is our hope that the information and strategies presented in this book will assist you to adopt and implement the best methods we know of to date to help our children be safe and productive in their schooling experience.

Contents

List of Tables, Figures,
Boxes, and Forms

TABLES

FIGURES

BOXES

FORMS

1

At-Risk Youth and School Safety

Critical Issues, Current Challenges, and Promising Approaches

In the last decade of the 20th century, the United States and its public schools were profoundly shaken by a series of school shooting tragedies that changed the landscape of school security and destroyed, perhaps forever, the sense of relative safety that students, families, and educators have traditionally held about the schooling process and the physical setting in which it occurs. All who are concerned with the schooling of our vulnerable children and youth were powerfully affected by these terrible events. Even though schools, compared to other social contexts, are one of the safest places for our children and youth (Kingery & Walker, 2002), school settings are no longer regarded by our society as exclusively safe havens in which students are free to develop academically and socially, unburdened by concern for their personal safety. In the wake of the school shootings in the mid to late 1990s, students and parents were traumatized on a broad scale by fears of school tragedies and concerns about lack of school security.

Jonesboro, Arkansas marked a watershed event in the history of school shootings. The safety of the Jonesboro school was shattered by an act of domestic terrorism planned and carried out by two young students who attended the school. These youth arranged for a fire alarm to be set off and then shot at teachers and students from outside the building as they vacated the school. Many adult and child victims were killed and wounded.

Many of the school shooting tragedies that followed Jonesboro were similar in type and scope, and their cumulative effect was to alter permanently the nature of

Portions of the material contained in this chapter were included in Walker (1996).

schooling in relation to issues of school security and student safety. The total number of students killed and wounded on school grounds in the decade of the 1990s was close in number to those in earlier decades. However, the magnitude and impact of the tragedies that occurred during the latter half of the last decade tended to be qualitatively different in terms of the following factors:

1. The number of killed and wounded per episode or tragedy
2. The randomness by which victims were selected as targets
3. The careful planning and conspiratorial nature of these school shootings
4. The use of school shootings as an instrument in settling scores for grievances, real or imagined

Because these features usually characterize terrorist acts, the general salience of these tragedies rose to unprecedented levels of concern and outrage in our society.

In particular, the tragedies of Columbine in Colorado and Thurston High School in Springfield, Oregon, stand out in this regard: They reflected a dedicated commitment by seriously disturbed high school students to redressing their grievances through revenge-seeking actions aimed at innocent parents, students, and school personnel. The shock, grief, and outrage that followed the tragedies of Thurston and Columbine galvanized the government into taking a series of dramatic actions geared toward improving school safety. One of these actions was the creation of the Early Warning/Timely Response document (Dwyer, Osher, & Warger, 1998) to assist schools in the enhancement of their overall safety. This document, jointly sponsored by the U.S. Departments of Justice and Education, was produced by a 25-member panel of experts that included the authors of this volume. All 125,000 public and private U.S. schools received a copy of Early Warning/Timely Response during the fall of 1998. In a related action the U.S. Department of Education funded the Safe Schools/Healthy Students initiative at the end of the decade, which provided funding support for school district–community collaborations to implement comprehensive programs that promote school safety. Over 150 grants were awarded as part of this initiative in three rounds of funding, and additional funding is still available. Finally, recent analyses of the characteristics of school shooters by the U.S. Secret Service (Fein et al., 2002) and a "threat assessment" protocol developed by the Federal Bureau of Investigation (FBI) provide information aimed at helping school personnel assess the level of risk presented by student threats or dangerous behavior. These actions have raised awareness of the factors that contribute to a lack of school safety and stimulated a broad range of protective activities by schools and communities.

Collectively, we have extensive experience as researchers, consultants, program developers, staff trainers, and policy experts in school safety and prevention of antisocial behavior. The Institute on Violence and Destructive Behavior (IVDB), in which we are principal investigators, was founded in 1994 at the University of Oregon to serve as a resource to school districts and other agencies in the area of school safety. Currently, the IVDB maintains a diverse portfolio of school safety activities and is the administering unit for numerous competitively awarded federal and state grants to support these activities. The IVDB and its key personnel serve as a research unit on behalf of school districts and also as a filter or evaluation vehicle to distinguish school safety information that is reliable and trustworthy from that which is not valid or even dangerous. The IVDB currently serves as the mandated Center for School Safety for the state of Oregon, as directed by the Oregon legislature, the state attorney general, and the governor, and as enacted in August 2001.

While recognizing that no school can ever be made perfectly safe, we believe that school safety is best conceptualized as a bipolar dimension (see Figure 1.1) that ranges

Unsafe Schools

(Lack of cohesion, chaotic classrooms, stress, disorganization, poor structure, ineffective administration, high-risk gang activity, violent incidents, unclear behavioral and academic expectations.)

Safe Schools

(Effective structure and organization; freedom from potential physical and psychological harm, absence of violence; presence of nurturing, caring, and protective staff)

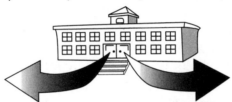

School-Based Risk Factors

- Poor design and use of school space
- Overcrowding
- Lack of caring but firm disciplinary procedures
- Insensitivity to, and poor accommodation of, multicultural factors
- Student alienation
- Rejection of at-risk students by teachers and peers
- Anger and resentment at school routines and demands for conformity
- Poor supervision

School-Based Protective Factors

- Positive school climate and atmosphere
- Clear and high performance expectations for *all* students
- Inclusionary values and practices throughout the school
- Strong student bonding to the school environment
- High levels of student participation and parent involvement in schooling
- Provision of opportunities for skill acquisition and social development
- Schoolwide conflict-resolution strategies

FIGURE 1.1. Bipolar dimensions and attributes of unsafe and safe schools, with associated risk and protective factors.

from unacceptable to acceptable. The dimension of school safety should not be thought of in absolute terms such as safe *or* unsafe but rather in comparative terms as *safer* versus *less safe*. It is the responsibility of school leaders to do all in their power to maximize the safety and security of their schools. As the social conditions (e.g., family and community environments) in the neighborhoods served by many individual schools continue to deteriorate, the challenge for educators of maintaining acceptable school safety levels grows ever more difficult and requires the investment of greater and greater resources that would otherwise be allocated to the positive social and academic development of students.

The goal of this resource book is to bring state-of-the-art information and empirically supported practices to the process of making schools safer. The following topics are addressed within this chapter: (1) school safety and security; (2) antisocial behavior, delinquency, and youth violence; (3) current status and trends in youth violence and school safety; (4) conceptualizing school safety; (5) sources of vulnerability to school safety; (6) assessing school safety; (7) what the science says about what does and does not work in school crime prevention; and (8) school safety intervention strategies.

SCHOOL SAFETY AND SECURITY

Box 1.1 provides statistics on school safety that document how our schools have changed over the past two decades. These statistics reflect some of the challenges now facing educators in the mass processing of an increasingly diverse population of

---

BOX 1.1. Statistics on School Safety

- Over 100,000 students bring weapons to school each day, and 40 students are killed or wounded with these weapons annually.

- Large numbers of students fear victimization on the way to and from school, where bullies and gang members are likely to prey on them.

- Twenty-two percent of students in our nation's schools are afraid to use school bathrooms because these relatively unsupervised areas are often sites for assaults and others forms of serious victimization.

- More than 6,000 teachers are threatened annually, and well over 200 are physically injured by students on school grounds.

- Increasingly, students are intimidated and threatened by the mean-spirited teasing, bullying, and sexual harassment that occur at school.

- Schools often serve as major sites for the recruitment activities of organized gangs.

school-age children and youth. They also indicate that the safety and well-being of students and adults in the school setting cannot be taken for granted any longer. Kingery and Walker (2002) reviewed what is currently known about school safety and used evidence-based knowledge to separate some of the myths from facts. These authors also addressed the issue of students carrying weapons on school grounds and methods for reducing this threat to school safety.

There is little doubt that the declining social conditions of our society have spilled over into the process of schooling in very unfortunate ways. Thousands of students enter school with a history of exposure to multiple and overlapping risks (e.g., family dysfunction, drug and alcohol abuse by caregivers, abuse [physical, sexual, and emotional] at the hands of relatives and acquaintances, poverty, divorce, and domestic violence). Today's student population is flooded with exposure to risk factors that negatively impact students' lives at family, school, neighborhood, and community levels. The cumulative effect of these risks is to place vulnerable children and youth on a pathway to destructive outcomes in adolescence and young adulthood (e.g., drug and alcohol abuse, delinquency, violent acts, and criminal behavior). In the absence of offsetting protective factors or the ability to access key support services and structures, it is unlikely that these individuals will be able to get off this destructive path if it has not been accomplished by the end of the primary grades (Kazdin, 1993). Rather, these individuals will likely require ongoing support and services throughout their lives to reduce the harm they cause themselves and others.

It is very likely that not a single school in the United States has been unaffected by the changed landscape of school safety and security. Electronic and mechanical approaches that involve sophisticated technology to solving school security problems are now standard fare in many school settings, especially those serving urban areas (see Green, 1999). Crisis intervention planning and staff training for a potential school tragedy are now required elements in the operational procedures of many school districts and individual schools. Schools serving deteriorating urban communities and neighborhoods routinely employ public safety and school resource officers as part of the regular school staff; this practice is spreading rapidly to suburban communities as well. Violence prevention curricula are used routinely to teach anger management and conflict resolution skills to all students in thousands of today's schools. For example, the Second Step Violence Prevention Curriculum, developed by the Committee for Children (1993, 2002), is currently used in 15,000 U.S. schools.

Federal agencies, including the U.S. Office of Safe and Drug-Free Schools (now under the office of Homeland Security), have created expert panels to review and recommend intervention approaches that will enhance school safety. School officials are now open to preventive intervention approaches that were given scant attention just a few years ago. More ominously, enormous pressures are mounting among educators to profile potentially at-risk students and to identify those considered most likely to commit an act of school violence—even though acceptable and valid methods for accomplishing this goal remain obscure. With the exception of attempts to profile school shooters, the collective impact of these changes is generally positive in nature and has contributed to safer and more effective schools.

ANTISOCIAL BEHAVIOR, DELINQUENCY, AND YOUTH VIOLENCE

The overall juvenile crime rate and the alarming increase in interpersonal violence are associated with a dramatic escalation in the number of children who bring antisocial behavior patterns to the schooling experience (American Psychological Association, 1993; Loeber & Farrington, 1998b, 2001; Thornton, Craft, Dahlberg, Lynch, & Baer, 2000). In the past several decades, the number of children and families displaying antisocial behavior has surged significantly (Patterson, Reid, & Dishion, 1992; Reid, Patterson, & Snyder, 2002). The U.S. rate of interpersonal violence finally stabilized in 1992, after a decade of unprecedented increases (Satcher, 2001). Child delinquents (i.e., those who commit offenses prior to the age of 12) are now a major focus of concern by the U.S. Office of Juvenile Justice and Delinquency Prevention. Three of the four crimes (robbery, rape, and murder) used to construct the FBI's annual violence index have returned to levels prior to the huge surge that began in the early 1980s, fueled mainly by the crack-cocaine epidemic. However, aggravated assault levels have not shown such a reversal and remain a cause of great concern by policymakers, federal officials, and legislators concerned with juvenile crime issues (see Satcher, 2001). Figure 1.2, from the U.S. Surgeon General's 2001 report on youth violence (Satcher, 2001), illustrates trends in these indices over the past two decades.

Antisocial behavior provides a fertile breeding ground for the later development of a delinquent lifestyle. Indeed, antisocial behavior that (1) begins early in a child's life, (2) occurs across multiple settings and contexts, (3) is expressed in diverse forms, and (4) occurs at a high frequency is one of the best predictors we have of later juvenile crime (Reid, 1993). Loeber and Farrington (2001) argue that there is a well-established pathway from severe disruptive behavior that leads to child delinquency and culminates in adolescent delinquency. Furthermore, Coie (1994) notes that if children are antisocial at home *and* school, they are 50% more likely to be violent than if they are antisocial in only one of these settings. Schools are increasingly victimized by children and youth who are themselves victims of pervasive poverty, abuse, neglect, chaotic family environments, crime-ridden neighborhoods, racial discrimination, a sense of hopelessness, and so on (Soriano, 1994).

The American Psychological Association produced a superb synthesis of the knowledge base related to the prevalence of violence among youth and associated causal factors, and recommended approaches to addressing this violence (see American Psychological Association, 1993). This task force report contains important observations and recommendations that have considerable currency today (see Box 1.2).

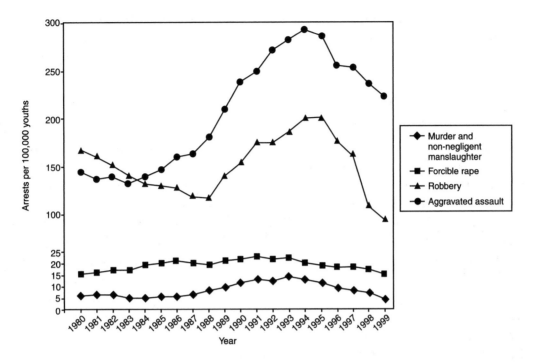

FIGURE 1.2. Arrest rates of youths ages 10–17 for serious violent crime, by type of crime, 1980–1999. From Satcher (2001).

**BOX 1.2. American Psychological Association Task Force Observations
on Youth and Violence**

1. Violence is not the human condition; it is learned behavior that is preventable.

2. Violence cuts across all lines of culture and ethnicity; it is not exclusive to any single group or class.

3. Prevention of violence requires education of and by all segments of society; it also requires a reassessment of how conflict is viewed and resolved.

4. There are four individual social experiences that contribute powerfully to the increase in violence among children and youth: easy access to firearms (especially handguns), early involvement with drugs and alcohol, association with antisocial groups, and pervasive exposure to violent acts portrayed in the media.

5. Schools must be a hub or key center of activity in the development of comprehensive, interagency interventions for the prevention and remediation of violent behavior.

The Oregon Social Learning Center (OSLC) has conducted some of the best cross-sectional and longitudinal research studies on family risk factors associated with children and youth who adopt antisocial behavior patterns that result in juvenile delinquency and adult criminal behavior (see Patterson et al., 1992; Reid et al., 2002). OSLC researchers have identified six key risk factors that are strongly associated with becoming a juvenile offender: (1) mother was arrested at some point in her adult life, (2) father was arrested at some point in his adult life, (3) family has documented involvement with child protective services, (4) at least one family transition (e.g., divorce) or death of a family member has occurred, (5) the child received special education services at one time or another, and (6) child displays early onset of antisocial behavior. OSLC analyses show that any combination of three of these factors puts the child or youth at substantial risk of becoming a repeat juvenile offender. Large numbers of youth who are referred by public safety officials to juvenile detention manifest these characteristics. The more of these risks a youth has in his or her life, the more likely recidivism is to occur in terms of delinquent acts committed following adjudication.

Within the context of schooling, McEvoy and Welker (2000) have analyzed the research knowledge base relating to academic underachievement, learning problems, and antisocial behavior. They make a persuasive case that the majority of failed attempts to make schools safer tend to have three negative characteristics in common: (1) they have failed to take into account the interrelationship that exists among these three dimensions (i.e., academic underachievement, learning problems, and antisocial behavior); (2) they have tended to focus on characteristics and attributes of individual students, to the exclusion of the known risk factors and conditions that are predictive of antisocial behavior and underachievement; and (3) they overlook the fact that school climate is a powerful variable in the mix of factors and needs to be addressed in the school safety agenda.

We strongly support these conclusions and are advocates of whole-school interventions that clearly communicate and enforce consistent behavioral expectations for all students and that create a climate of competence and mutual respect within the school setting. Examples of such programs include the Second Step Violence Prevention Curriculum (Frey, Hirschstein, & Guzzo, 2000), the School-Wide Positive Behavior Support (SWPBS) model (Horner, Sugai, Lewis-Palmer, & Todd, 2001), the best behavior staff development program (Sprague & Golly, 2004; Sprague et al., 2001), and the schoolwide ecological intervention, developed by Nelson and his colleagues (see Nelson, 2000). All of these interventions are empirically based and proven to work when assessed using both schoolwide measures as well as measures of individual student behavior. They are highly recommended to educators concerned with making schools safer.

Walker and his colleagues (Walker, Colvin, & Ramsey, 1995; Walker & McConnell, 1995b) have found the following three risk factors, if present in grade 5, to be highly predictive of arrests in grade 10, within a high-risk sample of males: (1) weak social skills, (2) a higher-than-normal frequency of within-school discipline referrals from teachers, and (3) a high rate of negative, aggressive behavior directed toward peers on the playground (i.e., more than 12% of the time observed). Similarly, Tobin, Sugai, and Colvin (1996) found that office referrals for discipline problems involving harassment or fighting in grade 6 was a reliable predictor of serious behavior problems in grade 8. Even one such referral in grade 6 was associated with deferred high school graduation. These risk factors allow us to identify for intervention those students who are likely to be unsuccessful in school, who may eventually drop out, and who are likely to be arrested one or more times for delinquent acts.

There is also an extensive knowledge base on the behavioral correlates of effective *teacher-related* and *peer-related* social–emotional adjustments that *all* children have to negotiate within the context of schooling. Students who fail to make either of these critically important adjustments are behaviorally at risk; those who fail both of them place their school success and overall life quality at risk (Walker, Irvin, Noell, & Singer, 1992; Walker et al., 1996). Figure 1.3 illustrates an interpersonal model of social–behavioral adjustment within the school setting that includes these two types of adjustment, the behavioral correlates that enhance and impair them, and the long-term outcomes associated with each.

These research outcomes and knowledge base indicate the broad range of progress that has been made in understanding the origins of antisocial behavior patterns, how they develop over the long term, and the risk and protective factors that account for them. However, the gap between what is known about intervening effectively with these problems and actual practice is far too wide and needs to be addressed. This is especially the case within the context of school safety. One of the goals of this book is to narrow that gap.

CURRENT STATUS AND TRENDS IN YOUTH VIOLENCE AND SCHOOL SAFETY

The following observations and facts regarding youth violence and school safety frame the process of schooling, as we begin the 21st century. They present enormous challenges for school leaders and administrators and call for access to the best, most reliable information available for making schools safer and violence free.

1. Results from a study by the U.S. Centers for Disease Control (Thornton et al., 2000) indicate that between July 1994 and June 1998 there were 188 violent deaths on or near school grounds or at school-associated events. A majority of these incidents

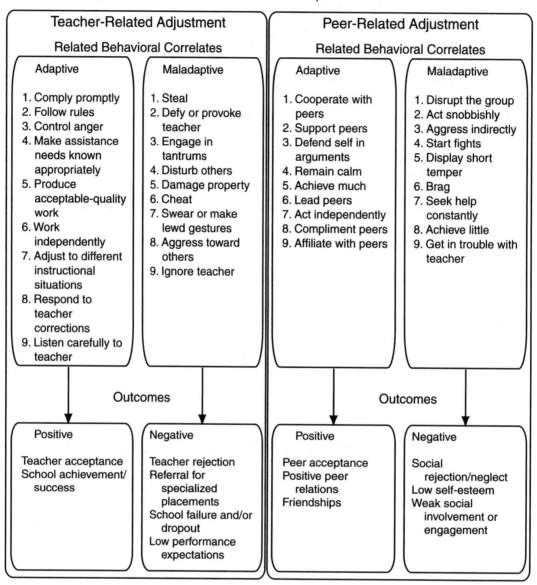

FIGURE 1.3. Model of interpersonal social–behavioral competence within school settings.

involved the use of firearms to commit homicides. The acts of violence occurred in communities of all sizes, ethnic/racial makeups, and geographic locations.

2. Much larger numbers of school tragedies would likely have occurred during this period, were it not for their prevention via early detection and disclosure by peers. More students who hear of plans for school violence are now reporting them to school authorities. The Ribbon of Promise (*www.ribbonofpromise.org*) and the SAVE (Students against Violence Everywhere) programs are two nationally known organizations that have been prominent in these student-led preventive efforts.

3. Each school shooting now produces a number of copycat incidents, suggesting that these events have been planned and contemplated for some time rather than spontaneously arising in connection with a tragedy.

4. The public and parents generally have moved beyond expressing concern for the troubled youth who commit these tragedies to voicing their outrage about them and making demands for ensuring that schools become safer for all children and youth.

5. Schools, students, and parents are now increasingly victimized by fears about the possibility of a tragedy occurring in their particular setting. Such pervasive fear lowers overall quality of life and reduces students' ability to get the most out of the schooling process.

6. The societal forces that infiltrate the schooling process and are associated with these tragedies include dysfunctional families, incivility, substance abuse, child neglect and abuse, the flood of media violence, the anger and social fragmentation that are pervasive in our society, and so on. These forces have been developing for a long time and will not change or vanish in the near term.

7. A major concern vis à vis school tragedies is today's peer culture. Increasingly, our youth are immersed in a peer culture that is coarse, crude, cruel, uncaring, and often destructive to an individual's self-esteem.

8. Bullying, sexual harassment, and mean-spirited teasing are normative processes in many school settings and poison their climates. These destructive processes are often encouraged and supported by the presence and attention of peer bystanders.

   a. An estimated 160,000 students miss school every day in the United States because of bullying and threats of intimidation.
   b. Fully two-thirds of school shooters interviewed by the U.S. Secret Service were teased and bullied in their school careers.

It is remarkable that so many of today's youth are, in some instances, willing to "write off" the rest of their lives as a consequence of settling their grievances by using violence against their peers, teachers, and even parents. Many of these youth are very likely suicidal, extremely depressed, and in urgent need of mental health services and support. At-risk students who hold these views and manifest these characteristics are at severe risk to themselves as well as to key social agents in their lives. In addition, they can represent a serious threat to the safety of the entire school population.

CONCEPTUALIZING SCHOOL SAFETY

Schools are highly vulnerable to interpersonal violence and gang activity. Furlong and Morrison (1994, 2000) have reframed the issue of school violence within a conceptual model of school safety that (1) includes both developmental and educational concepts and (2) emphasizes prevention and schooling effectiveness. These authors argue that effectively dealing with school violence requires careful attention to a broad range of considerations regarding school safety; for example, schools that are violence free are also effective at teaching and evince a caring, nurturing, inclusive, achieving, and accepting environment. The absence of violence is but one element among a larger constellation of positive factors that characterize safe schools.

Figure 1.1 (p. 3) illustrates this conceptualization along a bipolar dimension that ranges from unsafe to safe. The relative safety of schools is represented in terms of the number and nature of the risk and protective factors that are present. As with individuals, risk factors and conditions move the school in the direction of less safety. The greater the number of risk factors/conditions, the more powerful they are, and the longer they are in evidence, the greater their destructive impact on the school's safety. Protective factors, as listed in this figure, have the potential to buffer, offset, and reduce the destructive impact of risk conditions on the school's status and operation. Schools can be distributed along this dimension in terms of performance indicators that document how relatively safe or unsafe they are: for example, the number of victimization instances, levels of supervision, academic achievement levels, number of disciplinary referrals per student and for the whole school, the nature of the school's social climate, the presence or absence of gang activity, and so on. A reliable composite index of these measures could be developed and used to locate an individual school along this dimension.

SOURCES OF VULNERABILITY TO SCHOOL SAFETY

Major sources of vulnerability to school safety and security have been described and analyzed by Sprague et al. (2002). These authors regard the following areas as potentially vulnerable to significant threats to the safety and security of schools: (1) the design, use, and supervision of school space, (2) the administrative and management practices of the school, (3) the nature of the neighborhood and community served by the school, and (4) the characteristics of the students enrolled. Figure 1.4 illustrates these four areas and provides indicators of each type of school safety vulnerability. If an individual school registers a positive profile across these dimensions, it is much more likely to experience acceptable levels of safety and security than if it registers a negative profile, where many risk factors are in evidence. We believe that any compre-

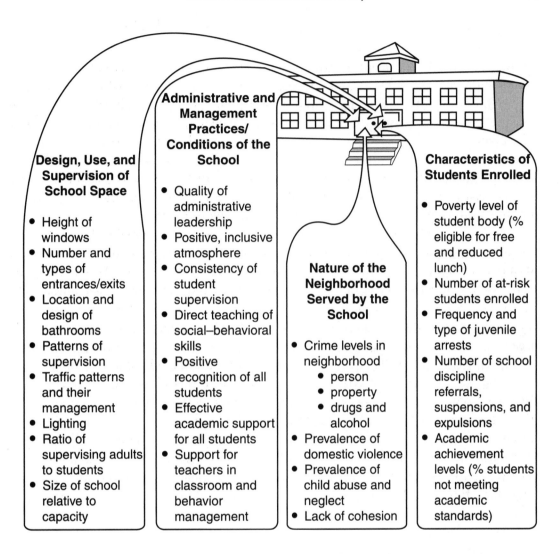

FIGURE 1.4. Four sources of vulnerability to school safety.

hensive approach to ensuring a school's safety should evaluate and address these dimensions of risk. Chapter 2 provides additional information regarding these four areas or potential sources of risk and recommends the use of specific assessment tools.

The architectural design and operation of school space can be an important source of vulnerability to a school's overall safety. For example, the number of unlocked and unmonitored entrances to the school, the nature and amount of supervision available for low-traffic areas, the location of bathrooms, the ability of school personnel to easily provide "natural" surveillance of school grounds, and the size of hallways that are typically crowded with students during certain periods of the day—all are examples of areas vulnerable to threats to school safety. These areas, when found vulnerable, require architectural retrofitting and/or allocation of staff resources. The knowledge base relating to school design and retrofitting to enhance school safety comes from the important work of experts in Crime Prevention through Environmental Design (CPTED; see Crowe, 1991). A thorough treatment of this topic is contained in Schneider, Walker, and Sprague (2000). Some of the topics addressed in this volume include a description of key CPTED concepts and principles, the relevance of CPTED as a strategy for improving school safety and security, school-site CPTED evaluation procedures, case-study applications of CPTED principles, the role of architects in school design, and CPTED-based policy recommendations for consideration by school districts.

The administrative and management practices of the school's leadership have a tremendous influence on the social climate of the school. As noted earlier, McEvoy and Welker (2000) have reviewed the research on this important dimension and argue that school climate must be fully addressed to make schools safer and more academically effective. Research indicates that safer schools tend to be more effective schools, and vice versa (see Furlong & Morrison, 1994). The more recent analysis by McEvoy and Welker certainly confirms this finding. All students should perceive themselves as accepted and valued members of the school population; as fully able to participate in the extracurricular activities of the school; and as free from bullying, mean-spirited teasing, discrimination, or harassment. It is of critical importance that at-risk students who are socially marginalized and/or show signs of depression or other serious mental health problems receive the appropriate services and types of support. Students who leave school before graduating often indicate that they did not feel accepted in their school environment and that no one seemed to care about them or their problems.

The neighborhoods and communities served by schools can, and usually do, have a direct influence on the nature of the school and its overall safety. Schools that serve neighborhoods with high frequencies of police calls, street crime, poverty, unsupervised youth, and deteriorating infrastructure and buildings are much more likely to be unsafe than those whose attendance areas do not have these characteristics. It has been said that an individual school can be no safer than the neighborhoods and communities it serves. This statement may or may not hold true, depending on the nature of the social and environmental conditions under which the school operates. For example, some schools located in chaotic and dangerous urban environs are fortress-like structures that do appear to be safer than their surrounding neighborhoods. Whenever possible, schools should be integrated into the communities they serve and be viewed as partners with the other local agencies that serve children, youth, and families. However, when violence and serious crime are common occurrences in proximal neighborhoods, realizing this goal may be difficult. In such situations, schools have very few options by which they can attempt to improve the safety of the neighborhoods and communities they serve.

The fourth source of vulnerability in Figure 1.4 is the overall profile of the students who comprise the student body: poverty level; number of at-risk students; frequency and type of juvenile arrests; number of school referrals, suspensions, and expulsions; and academic achievement levels. These dimensions determine, to a very large extent, how students behave in school and whether they display rule-governed forms of behavior. This vulnerability source provides the most direct avenue whereby the toxic conditions of our society infiltrate and disrupt the process of schooling. Students who come from highly at-risk backgrounds and experience chaos and family dysfunction on a daily basis typically reflect these influences in how they behave in the school context. Too often, the resulting consequences are negative for the individual as well as the school environment.

The majority of attempts to make schools safe have focused on the student population and its behavioral characteristics. Although student behavior can pose a major risk to school safety, it is important to be aware that any comprehensive and successful school safety effort also must address the other three sources of vulnerability. The next section provides information and guidelines about how to assess a school's relative safety and to recognize the danger signs early in the risk-escalation process.

ASSESSING SCHOOL SAFETY

There are two dimensions of school safety that every school should consider. One involves the overall safety of the school building and grounds. That is, relative to normative standards, as defined by schools in general, how secure is the setting from victimization by violence, vandalism, gang activity, and so on? The other equally important dimension of school safety involves the social environment of the school in relation to the risk factors that reduce safety and the protective factors that enhance it. It is important that schools consider strategies for assessing these two dimensions of safety at least annually. Some recommended strategies and instruments for conducting these assessments are described briefly below.

To address the first dimension of school safety, the National School Safety Center has developed the School Crime Assessment Tool. A copy of this 20-item instrument is contained in Form 1.1 at the end of the chapter. Permission to reproduce and use it can be obtained from the National School Safety Center, Suite 290, 4165 Thousand Oaks Boulevard, Westlake Village, CA 91362. Each "yes" answer to the questions on this scale is assigned a value of 5 points. The scale can be completed by the school principal, a schoolwide teacher-assistance team, or a site-based management council. Total score on this instrument provides an estimate of the overall status of the school on the dimension of school safety. A score of 70 or more indicates very serious school safety problems; a score of 50 or more suggests the existence of significant problems in this area. A score between 25 and 45 indicates the need to develop a school safety plan. This simple measure provides a quick and easy estimate of a school's relative safety and should be considered as a first step to address the issue of school safety.

Relative to the social environment of the school and the specific risk and protective factors that impact it, the Institute on Violence and Destructive Behavior (IVDB) has developed the Oregon School Safety Survey (OSSS; Sprague, Colvin, Irvin, & Stieber, 1997a). A copy of this instrument is contained in Form 1.2 at the end of the chapter. Permission to use it can be obtained by contacting the first author of this book at the Institute on Violence and Destructive Behavior, 1265 University of Oregon, Eugene, OR 97403.

The OSSS describes 17 risk factors (those that increase the chance of violence and reduce school safety) and 16 protective factors (those that buffer the school against violence and enhance safety). These items were based on a review of the literature on violence prevention and crisis management in schools (e.g., Furlong & Morrison, 1994, 2000). Each item is rated on a 5-point scale that estimates the extent to which the risk or protective factor exists.

The purpose of this instrument is to assist educators in evaluating (1) the extent to which the school provides a safe learning environment, (2) training and support needs related to school safety and violence prevention, and (3) responses to school safety and violence by school staff. The survey is divided into three sections. Section One identifies the school's status regarding the major risk factors associated with school safety and violence. Section Two lists common protective factors and existing response plans to address school safety and violence concerns. Section Three provides respondents with an opportunity to make narrative comments regarding school safety and violence prevention. Five questions are provided to elicit open-ended comments.

Under the auspices of the statewide Confederation of School Administrators, the survey was distributed to a large sample of elementary, middle, and high school principals in Oregon. Usable data were obtained from 346 returned surveys representing a similar number of Oregon schools. Detailed results are described in Sprague, Colvin, Irvin, and Stieber (1997b). Preliminary analyses of this data base indicated that the instrument has excellent psychometric characteristics. The survey results (i.e., rankings of the relative importance of risk and protective factors) varied, as would be predicted, across elementary, middle, and high schools. Further studies of OSSS psychometrics and normative levels are planned by investigators within the IVDB. In addition, use of the instrument as a basis for developing safe school plans will be evaluated as part of this continuing effort.

BOX 1.3. Recommendations for Creating and Maintaining Safe Schools

- Regularly review Board of Education policies with school staff regarding pupil safety and protection, pupil discipline, and staff responsibilities.
- Discuss school crisis intervention plans with all staff and volunteers.
- Set up a staff supervision assignment map of the school that focuses on entrances, exits, and problem areas.
- Enlist formal and informal student leaders, staff, and parents to communicate student behavior and dress code expectations (e.g., direct teaching, intercom announcements, student and parent letters, newsletters, posted signs).
- Maintain a zero tolerance for weapons, threats, intimidation, fighting, and other acts of violence.
- Post signs requiring all visitors to sign in and out at the office and to obtain a visitor/volunteer button or ID card.
- Train and encourage all staff to personally contact visitors and refer them to the office.
- Minimize the number of unlocked entrances; post signs referring people to main unlocked entrances.
- Have volunteer and staff teams monitor entrances, exits, and halls for students and visitors.
- Require students to have a hall pass when moving about the school during class sessions.

Source: Satcher (2001).

WHAT THE SCIENCE SAYS ABOUT WHAT DOES AND DOES NOT WORK IN SCHOOL CRIME PREVENTION

The contributions of the Gottfredsons and their colleagues in the area of school safety and effectiveness represent very solid work on the identification of evidence-based strategies that work as well as those strategies and approaches that either do not work or actually worsen conditions. These researchers have studied national samples of schools to identify the factors, conditions, and characteristics that make them safer and more instructionally effective (see Gottfredson, 1997; Gottfredson, Gottfredson, & Czeh, 2000). Their work is highly recommended as a trustworthy and reliable source of information on this topic. Table 1.1 lists the generic strategies they recommend as effective and those that are considered to be ineffective.

We believe that the recommendations provided in Boxes 1.3 and 1.4 are useful and practical in addressing school safety issues and in reducing youth violence. Box 1.3

TABLE 1.1. Scientific Conclusions Regarding What Is and Is Not Effective in School Crime Prevention

What works?

Strategies for which at least two studies found positive effects on measures of problem behavior and for which the preponderance of evidence is positive are:

Crime and delinquency

- Programs aimed at building school capacity to initiate and sustain innovation.
- Programs aimed at clarifying and communicating norms about behavior by establishing school rules, improving the consistency of their enforcement (particularly when they emphasize positive reinforcement of appropriate behavior), or communicating norms through schoolwide campaigns (e.g., anti-bullying campaigns) or ceremonies.
- Comprehensive instructional programs that focus on a range of social competency skills (e.g., developing self-control, stress-management, responsible decision-making, social problem-solving, and communication skills) and that are delivered over a long period of time to reinforce those skills.

What does not work?

Strategies for which at least two studies found no positive effects on measures of problem behavior and for which the preponderance of evidence is not positive are:

- Counseling students, particularly in a peer-group context, does not reduce delinquency or substance abuse.
- Offering youths alternative activities, such as recreation and community service, in the absence of more potent prevention programming does not reduce substance use.
- Instructional programs focusing on information dissemination, fear arousal, moral appeal, and affective education are ineffective for reducing substance use.

What is promising?

In one rigorous study, several strategies have been shown to reduce delinquency or substance use. When the preponderance of evidence for these strategies is positive, they are regarded as "promising" until replication confirms the effect. These strategies are:

Crime and delinquency

- Programs that group youth into "schools-within-schools" to create smaller units, more supportive interactions, or greater flexibility in instruction.
- Behavior modification programs and programs that teach "thinking skills" to high-risk youths.
- Programs aimed at building school capacity to initiate and sustain innovation.
- Programs that improve classroom management and that use effective instructional techniques.

Note. From Gottfredson (1997).

BOX 1.4. Recommendations for Interventions, Conditions,
and Programs That Reduce Youth Violence

- Provide early childhood interventions in the form of extensive support services and training to teach all families, child-care and health-care providers how to deal with early childhood aggression.
- Provide developmentally appropriate school-based interventions in classroom management, problem solving, and violence prevention.
- Demonstrate sensitivity to issues of cultural diversity through community involvement in the development of violence prevention efforts.
- Advocate for mass media cooperation with the social responsibility to both limit the depiction of violence during child-viewing hours and educate children about violence prevention efforts.
- Advocate for the limitation of firearm accessibility to youth and the provision of firearm violence prevention training.
- Advocate for measures and programs that foster a reduction of alcohol and other drug use among youth.
- Provide ample mental health services for perpetrators, victims, and witnesses of violence.
- Provide prejudice-reduction programs that defuse hate crimes.
- Advocate for mob violence prevention efforts from police and community leaders.
- Demonstrate individual and professional commitment from the psychology community to reduce youth violence.

Source: American Psychological Association (1993).

BOX 1.5. Six Major Strategies for Promoting Safe and Healthy Schools

- Secure the school.
- Develop a comprehensive school safety and crisis-response plan.
- Create a positive, inclusive school climate and culture.
- Address the peer culture and its problems.
- Involve parents in making the school safer.
- Support at-risk and antisocial youth.

contains recommendations for safe schools, and Box 1.4 contains recommendations relating to youth violence. These recommendations are based on best practices, and the available evidence supports their application in today's schools.

SCHOOL SAFETY INTERVENTION STRATEGIES

In March 2001, Oregon's attorney general released the report of the Oregon School Safety Coalition on the level of safety present in Oregon's schools. This coalition assessed the landscape of school safety over a 15-month period and issued a report to guide school policies in this area. The report, which contains specific recommendations for increasing school safety, provided the foundation for school safety legislation that established the Oregon School Safety Center. This document is highly recommended as a resource for school administrators in Oregon; it can be downloaded from the IVDB website at *darkwing.uoregon.edu/~ivdb/*.

In our view, six strategic approaches have the potential to move schools in the direction of greater safety and reduce the likelihood, over time, of a school tragedy erupting. We recommend these generic strategies based on (1) our collective experience in developing interventions for educators to address the needs and problems of at-risk student populations; (2) our analysis of the professional literature and knowledge base on making schools safer and preventing school violence; and (3) our considerable experience in serving as independent evaluators for school safety projects implemented by school districts, in collaboration with mental health and public safety agencies and funded by the Safe Schools/Healthy Students Initiative. These strategies are outlined in Box 1.5 (page 19) and elaborated below.

The more at-risk a school is perceived to be, the more important and relevant these strategies become and the greater the investment required. Furthermore, their relevance and importance increase from elementary to middle to high school settings.

Secure the School

The most immediate and direct method of addressing school safety issues is to secure the school. The three primary approaches to consider seriously in this regard are (1) the appropriate use of school security technology, (2) employment of school resource officers, and (3) use of CPTED principles and techniques. Applied in combination, these three approaches can be effective in reducing the probability of a school shooting tragedy. Currently, the second and third approaches are built into the federally funded Safe Schools/Healthy Students initiative being implemented in many school districts across the country. Considerable progress has been made in the development and appropriate use of security technology to make schools safer without turning them

---

Box 1.6. Key Elements of Safe Schools Plans

Most states now have a law that requires each school to develop a *School Improvement Plan*. Given the changes in our society and youth population that have occurred over the past several decades, it is imperative that careful consideration be given by schools to developing a *Safe Schools Plan*. The key elements that should be addressed in a comprehensive school safety plan are as follows:

- School safety audits that evaluate school safety and violence vulnerabilities due to structural characteristics of the building and patterns of building usage.
- A crisis intervention plan that allows school personnel to respond to and control crises that carry potential implications for violence or reduced school safety.
- A schoolwide curricular program that teaches social skills instrumental in violence prevention (anger management, conflict resolution, empathy, and impulse control).
- A well-established communication plan that provides interactive linkages between school personnel, public safety, and parents.

These four elements would be essential to improving the safety and security of any school building and grounds. Well-developed procedures exist for assessing a school's degree of risk and for implementing each of the components listed above.

---

into fortress-like structures. This technology is also being used increasingly in schools across the country. An excellent resource on this topic has been developed and published by the U.S. Office of Juvenile Justice and Delinquency Prevention (see Green, 1999). School administrators should be aware of the status, advantages, and limitations of this technology when considering implementation of school safety options and strategies.

Develop a Comprehensive School Safety and Crisis-Response Plan

We believe that each state should mandate development of a written school safety and crisis-response plan. In today's social environment, it is essential that each school go through a planning process designed to reduce the likelihood of a school tragedy and to manage a crisis effectively if it occurs. Box 1.6 contains guidelines and key elements that should be considered in developing such plans. Paine and Sprague (2002) have identified steps for constructing a school safety and crisis-response plan and provides examples of each element that should go into such a plan.

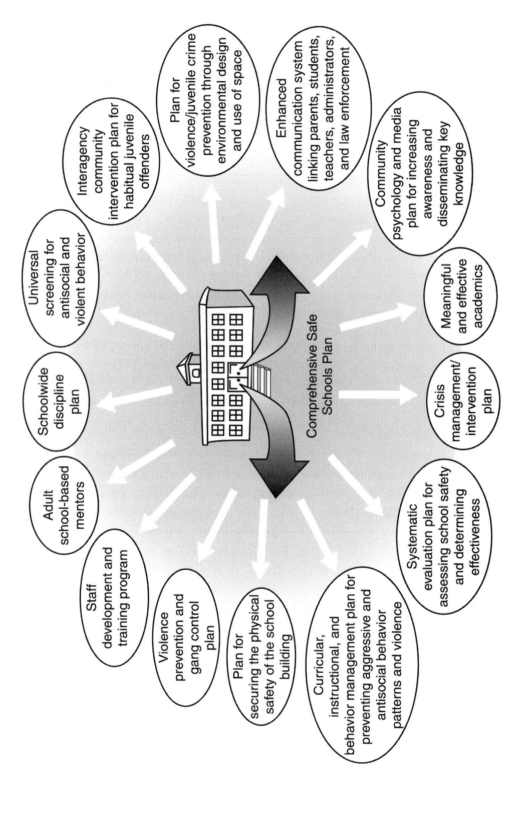

FIGURE 1.5. Major components of a prototype safe schools plan.

Plan for violence/juvenile crime prevention through environmental design and use of space

Enhanced communication system linking parents, students, teachers, administrators, and law enforcement

Interagency community intervention plan for habitual juvenile offenders

Community psychology and media plan for increasing awareness and disseminating key knowledge

Universal screening for antisocial and violent behavior

Meaningful and effective academics

Schoolwide discipline plan

Comprehensive Safe Schools Plan

Crisis management/ intervention plan

Adult school-based mentors

Systematic evaluation plan for assessing school safety and determining effectiveness

Staff development and training program

Violence prevention and gang control plan

Plan for securing the physical safety of the school building

Curricular, instructional, and behavior management plan for preventing aggressive and antisocial behavior patterns and violence

Figure 1.5 illustrates the key components of a prototype safe schools plan. These are the components that must be addressed effectively to ensure a safe school environment in today's society. The investment of effort and resources needed to create and enact these components will vary by school site and neighborhood. The higher the crime-risk status of the neighborhoods served by a particular school, the less safe that school is likely to be and the greater the effort and resources that will be required. Regardless of the degree of risk that exists, individual schools can systematically assess and address a number of risk and protective factors as part of an overall school safety enhancement plan (see earlier section on Assessing School Safety, pp. 15–16).

Create a Positive, Inclusive School Climate and Culture

As noted earlier, there is solid evidence that instructionally effective schools tend to be safer schools, and vice versa. The research of Gottfredson (1997; Gottfredson et al., 2000) and others shows that a school climate that is positive, inclusive, and accepting is a key component of an effective school. Three recommended strategies for addressing this component of school safety follow.

1. Create and promote a set of school-based positive values about how we treat others that include *civility, caring, and respect for the rights of others*.

It is unfortunate that teachers have to teach civility, in addition to everything else they do, but such is now the case. Children and youth are daily exposed to very poor adult models of uncivil behavior. Making civility a core value of the school's culture may help reduce some of the coarseness of the peer culture that has become such a problem in our schools and society.

2. Teach all students how to separate from their own lives the exaggerated media images of interpersonal violence, disrespect, and incivility to which they are exposed daily.

School curricula exist that teach media literacy relative to interpersonal violence. It is especially important that young children learn how to deconstruct the difference between media displays of violence and their own behavior and actions.

3. Establish and broadly communicate schoolwide rules and behavioral expectations and identify specific applications of them (i.e., in classrooms, hallways, lunchroom, playground, bus loading area).

It is important to consider whole-school approaches in dealing with the challenges of youth violence prevention and school safety/security issues. Too often, there is a singular focus on the most serious student offenders without a concomitant plan for addressing the potential needs and problems of the full population of students in the school. Such an inclusive plan would ultimately serve to prevent or reduce serious offenses. Whole-school approaches can change the climate of a school building and reduce the likelihood that the problems characteristically presented by at-risk students will escalate out of control (see Sprague, Sugai, & Walker, 1998; Walker et al., 1996).

The SWPBS approach is an excellent and proven vehicle for accomplishing this goal (Horner et al., 2001). Broadly implemented in school districts in Oregon and across the country, SWPBS is a highly recommended approach for schools to use in creating orderly, positive, and well-managed environments. Chapter 3 provides a comprehensive description of this approach and its intended outcomes.

Address the Peer Culture and Its Problems

The primary target for our prevention and safer-schools efforts should be the peer culture. The norms, actions, beliefs, and values within broad sectors of today's peer culture are socially destructive and demeaning. Many youth experience a "trial by fire" in negotiating the complex and difficult social tasks involved in finding their place in this peer culture. Far too many fail this critical test, become lost within it, and wander aimlessly while seeking an acceptance that is generally not forthcoming. They become homeless persons within the larger peer group and their lack of fit is well known. This painful reality forces many marginalized youth to affiliate with atypical or deviant peer groups, which can prove highly destructive for them.

Transforming this destructive peer culture is perhaps our most formidable task in the area of school safety. This culture is not of the school's making, but schools, collectively, comprise perhaps the only social institution, excluding the family, that is capable of addressing it effectively. Five ongoing strategies are recommended for consideration in this regard.

1. *Adopt and implement the Ribbon of Promise school violence prevention programs. By Kids, For Kids (BK4K), Not My Friends, Not My School, and Students against Violence Everywhere (SAVE) all involve students as key partners in making schools safe and violence free.*

These programs are designed to transform peer attitudes and beliefs about the risks to school safety that emerge from their culture. They promote peer ownership of the tasks involved in preventing school tragedies and are highly recommended as a first strategy for enlisting a school's peer culture in this effort. The Ribbon of Promise videos have been widely distributed and are available to schools nationally from their website at *www.ribbonofpromise.org*.

2. *Bully-proof the school setting by adopting effective anti-bullying/harassment programs, such as Bully Proofing Your School and Steps to Respect, which are available (respectively) from Sopris West, Inc., in Longmont, Colorado, at 303-651-2829,*

www.sopriswest.com; *and the Committee for Children in Seattle, at 800-634-4449,* www.cfchildren.org.

The best "disinfectant" for bullying, mean-spirited teasing, and harassment is sunlight—exposure. These events need to be defined as clearly unacceptable by everyone involved in the school (i.e., administrators, teachers, other school staff, students, and parents) and made public when they do occur. Students should be given strategies for reporting and coping with these events in an adaptive fashion. Furthermore, the reporting of those who commit these acts should be made acceptable. The programs cited above incorporate these basic principles and strategies.

3. *Teach anger-management and conflict-resolution techniques as part of regular curricular content.*

The Second Step Violence Prevention Curriculum, developed by the Committee for Children in Seattle (discussed in greater detail in Chapter 5), is one of the best means available for creating a positive peer culture of caring and civility and also for teaching specific strategies that work in controlling/managing anger and resolving conflicts without resorting to coercion or violence.

4. *Ask students to sign a pledge not to tease, bully, or put down others.*

Reports from schools that have tried this tactic indicate that it makes a difference in the number of incidents that occur and in the overall school climate.

5. *Refer troubled, agitated, and depressed youth to mental health services and ensure that they receive the professional attention they need.*

Involve Parents in Making the School Safer

With each new school shooting tragedy, parents of school-age children and youth seek greater assurances that their child's school is safe and, increasingly, are asking for a voice and role in helping the school attain this goal. Recently, a prosecuting attorney, the mother of four children, described a plan for creating a parent-based advocacy group on school safety that would rate the safety of schools and make this information available to all parents. Parents have much to offer in this regard and can be a powerful force in bringing greater safety and a sense of security to the school setting. The recently passed No Child Left Behind Act by Congress contains provisions for defining a persistently dangerous school. Parents of students in such schools can arrange to have them transferred to another school.

Four strategies are recommended for facilitating parent involvement in making a school safer:

1. *Create a parent advisory group devoted to school safety issues for that school.*
Such an advisory group would bring valuable knowledge, experience, and advocacy to the process of dealing with school-related safety challenges. It could also serve as a forum for reacting to district- and state-level policy directives in this area.

2. Advocate for parents to teach their children adaptive, nonviolent methods of responding to bullying, teasing, and harassment at school and to avoid encouraging them to "fight back."

In the vast majority of cases, fighting back is not effective and may escalate the situation to dangerous levels. Furthermore, it is more likely to increase the probability of the offensive behavior recurring rather than reducing it. A school-based anti-bullying program that has parental support and involvement is likely to be much more effective.

3. Advocate for the secure handling of weapons kept at home and for gun safety instruction for all family members.

Given the number of guns in U.S. homes, it is becoming imperative that everyone have some understanding of the dangers involved in handling guns and of being in proximity to those who are doing so. Trigger locks and secured gun cases are essential elements for storing weapons in the home, where the keys to same are also secured. The National Rifle Association has developed excellent information on gun safety that can be accessed by anyone. In connection with these efforts, young children need to be taught a "Golden Rule" about the sanctity of life and that guns are deadly, life-ending instruments.

4. Make available to parents solid information on effective parenting practices and provide access to parent training classes to those parents who seek additional guidance and support in their efforts to parent more effectively.

There are five generic parenting practices that are instrumental in determining how children develop: (1) discipline, (2) monitoring and supervision, (3) parent involvement in children's lives, (4) positive family-management techniques, and (5) effective crisis-intervention and problem-solving methods. A large number of available parent training programs address these parenting practices.

Support At-Risk Youth and Antisocial Youth

Youth with serious mental health problems and disorders who are alienated, socially rejected, and taunted by peers can be dangerous to themselves and others. These students are often well known to peers and staff in the school and should be given appropriate professional and parental attention, access to services, and social support. Severe bullying and taunting of students with mental health problems by peers has proven to be a dangerous combination in the context of potential school shootings.

CONCLUSION

We believe that Congress should consider passing legislation to regulate the exposure of children and youth to violent acts in the media and to develop family resource centers connected to school districts. Media violence is a subject of continuing controversy. There is considerable evidence that pervasive, long-term exposure to media violence (e.g., TV cartoons, video games, broadcast news, films, prime-time TV dramas) has two effects: (1) it desensitizes children and youth to violent acts, and (2) it makes individuals themselves more likely to commit violent acts (Hughes & Hasbrouck, 1996; Lieberman, 1994). These findings are especially applicable to behaviorally at-risk children and youth. Media violence serves as a social toxin that can poison the wellspring of our society. Parents must be informed about such effects on their children and how to attenuate them. Violent acts must be reduced and controlled "across the board" in the media. Curricula exist for assisting educators to teach children how to make sound judgments about, and interpretations of, what they are exposed to in the media (Hughes & Hasbrouck, 1996). These curricular approaches also inform children and youth about the negative effects that uncritical acceptance of this material can have on their lives.

Several states are experimenting with family resource centers connected to school districts (1) that allow parents to access support, assistance, and training, and (2) that also allow parents to deal with the school-related problems of their children in a nonjudgmental atmosphere. Such resource centers have great potential for creating the kind of partnerships necessary for parents and schools to work together as an effective team in making schools safer and creating more effective learning environments for all children, especially behaviorally at-risk students.

Punishing the at-risk student population and trying to exclude such students from schooling is not, by itself, an effective solution. For example, police indicate that 90% of daytime burglaries are committed by truant youth (Office of Juvenile Justice and Delinquency Prevention, 1993). Alternative programs and schools need to be developed for antisocial students, and we need to do far better in developing strategies for including them in mainstream educational processes. A therapeutic and habilitative school posture must be adopted, whenever possible, in dealing with this student population, and ways must be found to support and reclaim them. Powerful longitudinal research shows that school engagement, bonding, and success serve as protective factors in adolescence against a number of destructive outcomes, including violent delinquent acts, heavy drinking, teenage sex, and school dropout (Hawkins, Catalano, Kosterman, Abbott, & Hill, 1999).

Policy generally lags well behind the research that validates evidence-based approaches that can inform and guide regulations and practices based upon them. This is especially true in the area of school safety and violence prevention. The pressures and demands of the moment force school administrators into making decisions about school safety strategies and tactics that may appear promising but may not, as yet, be proven effective through the research process. Thus, we are left to choose among practices that appear promising, relying on our experience and using our best judgment, until the knowledge base on school safety becomes more solid, cohesive, evidence-based and widely used. The strategic actions described briefly above represent what we know about these complex issues at present. The material in the remainder of this volume fleshes out these strategies in forms that can be adopted and applied in today's school settings.

Historically, schools and school systems have remained comparatively detached players in the prevention of youth violence. Unfortunately, our society's problems have now spilled over into the process of schooling, so that ensuring school safety has emerged as a very high priority among parents of school-age children and youth (Soriano, 1994). Bullying, mean-spirited teasing, sexual harassment, and victimization are relatively commonplace occurrences on school campuses. Schools need to continue responding reactively to these crisis events as they occur. However, it is essential that they also begin investing in proactive, preventive approaches that will reduce the likelihood of future occurrences.

HOW THIS BOOK ADDRESSES THE RECOMMENDED STRATEGIES

This book is designed to assist school personnel to assess, select, and implement evidence-based school safety and prevention practices in today's schools. The content and recommendations herein are based on our experience assisting hundreds of schools across the United States (including seven of the federally funded Safe Schools/ Healthy Students communities), from our review of the literature on school safety and antisocial behavior, and from our own original research in the area. The remaining chapters are described briefly below.

• *Chapter 2: Developing a Comprehensive School Safety and Prevention Plan.* This chapter outlines a strategy that moves from comprehensive needs assessment to intervention selection to program evaluation. Recommended assessment tools and a framework for intervention selection are presented.

• *Chapter 3: Improving School Climate, Safety, and Student Health with Schoolwide Positive Behavior Supports.* Here we describe an integrated, sustainable system for implementing positive behavior support methods at the schoolwide level that is the foundation for all school safety approaches.

• *Chapter 4: Bullying and Peer-Based Harassment in Schools.* This chapter reviews the general characteristics, dynamics, and prevalence of the bully/victim problem in today's schools. It discusses legal and policy implications as well as methods for identifying bullies and their victims.

• *Chapter 5: Solutions for Bullying and Peer Harassment in the School Setting.* Here we outline strategies for preventing, ameliorating, and remediating the growing problem of bullying and peer harassment in our schools. Recommendations are provided for school personnel responsible for addressing bullying and harassment.

- *Chapter 6: Screening and Identifying Behaviorally At-Risk Students.* This chapter frames the critical issues and characterizes the landscape around early risk factors and the warning signs of potential violence. We describe recommended screening approaches in this area for use by school personnel. Access to this knowledge base is essential for every adult working in today's schools.

- *Chapter 7: Supporting Antisocial and Potentially Violent Youth.* Students who engage in antisocial and potentially violent behavior in school and other settings have complex and diverse support needs. These students often live amid circumstances known to predict life-course juvenile delinquency: for example, poverty, poor parental supervision, and crime-ridden neighborhoods. When not in school, these youth lack supervision and affiliate with other at-risk or already delinquent peers—circumstances that can easily lead to their involvement in juvenile crime. Given these circumstances, it is easy to understand why many behaviorally at-risk students experience serious adjustment problems that demand significant administrative time, disrupt regular classroom instruction, fail to respond to traditional school discipline, and, in some cases, pose a serious threat to the safety of other students or school staff. This chapter outlines a recommended approach for schools that is feasible and based on the best intervention research.

FORM 1.1. THE SCHOOL CRIME ASSESSMENT TOOL

The National School Safety Center has developed the following school-crime assessment tool to assist school administrators in evaluating their vulnerability to school-crime issues and potential school-climate problems.

1. Has your community crime rate increased over the past 12 months?   Yes ____ No ____

2. Are more than 15 percent of your work-order repairs vandalism related?   Yes ____ No ____

3. Do you have an open campus?   Yes ____ No ____

4. Has an underground student newspaper emerged?   Yes ____ No ____

5. Is your community transiency rate increasing?   Yes ____ No ____

6. Do you have an increasing presence of graffiti in your community?   Yes ____ No ____

7. Do you have an increased presence of gangs in your community?   Yes ____ No ____

8. Is your truancy rate increasing?   Yes ____ No ____

9. Are your suspension and expulsion rates increasing?   Yes ____ No ____

10. Have you had increased conflicts relative to dress styles, food services, and types of music played at special events?   Yes ____ No ____

11. Do you have an increasing number of students on probation in your school?   Yes ____ No ____

12. Have you had isolated racial fights?   Yes ____ No ____

13. Have you reduced the number of extracurricular programs and sports at your school?   Yes ____ No ____

14. Have parents increasingly withdrawn students from your school because of fear?   Yes ____ No ____

15. Has the budget for professional development opportunities and staff in-service training been reduced or eliminated?   Yes ____ No ____

16. Are you discovering more weapons on your campus?   Yes ____ No ____

17. Do you have written screening and selection guidelines for new teachers and other youth-serving professionals who work in your school?   Yes ____ No ____

18. Are drugs easily available in or around your school?   Yes ____ No ____

19. Are more than 40 percent of your students bused to school?   Yes ____ No ____

20. Have you had a student demonstration or other signs of unrest within the past 12 months?   Yes ____ No ____

(continued)

Permission to reproduce this form can be obtained from the National School Safety Center, Suite 290, 4165 Thousand Oaks Boulevard, Westlake Village, CA 91362.

Scoring and Interpretation

Multiply each affirmative answer by 5 and add the total.

0–20   Indicates no significant school safety problems.

25–45   An emerging school safety problem (safe-school plan should be developed).

50–70   Significant potential for school safety problem (safe-school plan should be developed).

Over 70 School is a sitting time bomb (safe-school plan should be developed immediately).

FORM 1.2. THE OREGON SCHOOL SAFETY SURVEY

Jeffrey R. Sprague, Geoffrey Colvin, and Larry K. Irvin
The Institute on Violence and Destructive Behavior
University of Oregon College of Education

Essential Questions for School Safety Planning

Please take a few minutes to complete the attached survey. Please place a check (✓) next to the item that best reflects your opinion for each question. Your responses will be valuable in determining training and support needs related to school safety and violence prevention.

Your Role:

Administrator ____   Related Service Provider ____
Teacher ____   Community Member ____
Special Education Teacher ____   Student ____
Parent ____   Other ____

Your School:

Elementary ____   High School ____
Middle/Junior High ____   Alternative School ____

Number of Students: Less than 500 ____   501–1,000 ____   More than 1,000 ____

Location: Rural ____
             Small Urban City (< 250,000) ____
             Large Urban City (> 250,000) ____

Section One: Assessment of Risk Factors for School Safety and Violence					
	Rating				
Indicate the extent to which these factors exist in your school and neighborhood:	Not at all	Minimally	Moderately	Extensively	Don't know
1. Illegal weapons.					
2. Vandalism.					
3. High student mobility (i.e., frequent changes in school enrollment).					

(continued)

FORM 1.2. *(page 2 of 4)*

	Not at all	Minimally	Moderately	Extensively	Don't know
4. Graffiti.					
5. Gang activity.					
6. Truancy.					
7. Student suspensions and/or expulsions.					
8. Students adjudicated by the court.					
9. Parents withdrawing students from school because of safety concerns.					
10. Child abuse in the home.					
11. Trespassing on school grounds.					
12. Poverty.					
13. Crimes (e.g., theft, extortion, hazing).					
14. Illegal drug and alcohol use.					
15. Fights, conflict, and assault.					
16. Incidence of bullying, intimidation, and harassment.					
17. Deteriorating condition of the physical facilities in the school.					

(continued)

Section Two: Assessment of Response Plans for School Safety and Violence Rating					
	Rating				
Indicate the extent to which these factors exist in your school and neighborhood:	Not at all	Minimally	Moderately	Extensively	Don't know
18. Opportunity for extracurricular programs and sports activities.					
19. Professional development and staff training.					
20. Crisis and emergency response plans.					
21. Consistently implemented schoolwide discipline plans.					
22. Student support services in school (e.g., counseling, monitoring, support team systems).					
23. Parent involvement in our school (e.g., efforts to enhance school safety, student support).					
24. Student preparation for crises and emergencies.					
25. Supervision of students across all settings.					
26. Suicide prevention/ response plans.					

(continued)

	Not at all	Minimally	Moderately	Extensively	Don't know
27. Student participation and involvement in academic activities.					
28. Positive school climate for learning.					
29. Acceptance of diversity.					
30. Response to conflict and problem solving.					
31. Collaboration with community resources.					
32. High expectations for student learning and productivity.					
33. Effective student– teacher relationships.					

Section Three: Your Comments on School Safety and Violence

1. What is the most pressing safety need in your school?

2. What school safety activities does your school do best?

3. What topics are most important for training and staff development?

4. What are the biggest barriers to improved school safety measures?

5. What other comments do you have regarding school safety?

6. What other factors not included in this survey do you believe affect school safety?

2

Developing a Comprehensive School Safety and Prevention Plan

with STEPHEN G. SMITH

BACKGROUND AND RATIONALE

Educators are provided a plethora of advice regarding effective school safety interventions but scant help in *integrating and sustaining* effective practices. We recommend that selection of interventions be based on a thorough assessment of the school's overall functioning (Sprague et al., 2002; Sugai, Lewis-Palmer, Todd, & Horner, 2000), with special attention given to disciplinary referral patterns (Sugai, Sprague, Horner, & Walker, 2000), self-reported violence perpetration and victimization (see Gottfredson, 1984; Boles, Biglan, & Smolkowski, 2003), and the security of the school building and grounds (Schneider, Walker, & Sprague, 2000). Thorough needs assessments in these areas (and others) can guide planning, avoid overlapping or conflicting services, and serve as the basis for the evaluation of change over time (Sprague et al., 2002).

Recommendations from the recent Surgeon General's report on school violence (Satcher, 2001; U.S. Department of Health and Human Services, 2001) provide a compelling rationale for adopting a prevention approach in which school is organized as a hub of intervention activities that focus on preventing the development of

Stephen G. Smith, MS, Institute on Violence and Destructive Behavior, College of Education, University of Oregon, Eugene, Oregon.

destructive antisocial peer networks and the reinforcement of deviancy. This report recommends that "an intolerant attitude toward deviance" be established by breaking up antisocial peer networks and changing the social climate of the school. Second, it recommends that we increase our "commitment to school" so that academic success is accessible to all children and positive school climates are established. Third, students should be taught and encouraged to display the skills and forms of behavior that enable them to respond appropriately to events that occasion and promote antisocial behavior.

This landmark report is buttressed by parallel recommendations in at least two other reports addressing the challenge of bringing effective interventions to scale. Mark Greenberg and his colleagues at Penn State University (Greenberg, Domitrovich, & Bumbarger, 1999) have outlined the research on effective, school-based interventions for antisocial behavior at the primary, secondary, and tertiary levels of prevention. We and others (see Gottfredson, 2001; Walker et al., 1996) recommend that schools attempt to offer integrated interventions at all three levels.

The challenge becomes how to give schools the capacity to adopt and sustain the processes, organizational structures, and systems that will enable them to carry out promising and proven interventions (Gottfredson, Gottfredson, & Czeh, 2000). The Gottfredsons recently conducted first-of-its-kind research (the National Study of Delinquency Prevention in Schools), and they argue convincingly that the problem is not the availability of *effective* programs (i.e., those that work), but rather it is one of *efficacy* (i.e., helping schools adopt and carry out the interventions and approaches in a manner that demonstrates effectiveness). It is likely that this problem of overlapping or poorly implemented intervention approaches is affected by a lack of useful needs assessment information and decision rules to guide the process.

Schools have always been judged by how well their students perform academically. Although destructive or violent behavior is a top concern and a direct influence on academic performance, systematic approaches to assessing schools on the basis of behavioral success or failure are not well developed at present. However, our schools are experiencing a strong push toward accountability on just that front.

Parents, schools, and community leaders need to make informed judgments about which systems are in place to prevent school violence and antisocial behavior. Title IV of the No Child Left Behind (NCLB) Act requires public schools to focus on the critical role of comprehensive needs assessment information in building and maintaining a school environment that is safe and conducive to learning.

In order to receive funds under Title IV, Part A, schools must adhere to the NCLB Principles of Effectiveness, as follows:

- Assess the specific safety risk and protective influences on the school.
- Establish measurable goals and objectives for improvement that are based on those identified needs.

- Base projected changes on appropriate measurements.
- Use evidence-based interventions for effecting improvement.

School safety plans must target what is required for the school to become safer and describe the activities or programs to be adopted that will address those targets. These activities and programs (1) must show research evidence of effectiveness in improving school safety, (2) involve parents in the assessment process, and (3) include performance measures to gauge effectiveness. In addition, each school district must have a comprehensive plan for school safety that includes policies, security procedures, prevention activities, crisis-response procedures, and a code of conduct for students that incorporates a "wrong and harmful" message about illegal drug use and violence. The plan needs to be made available to the public for review and comment.

Because of the importance of gathering and maintaining consistent data that provide a picture of how a school is performing, the new law requires school districts to monitor and report (1) truancy rates, (2) suspensions and expulsions related to drugs and violence, (3) the incidence, prevalence, and age of onset of alcohol use, drug use, and violence by youth (students are also to be asked about perceptions of health risks and social disapproval for use), and (4) incidents of criminal activity on school property.

This chapter provides a road map to success in achieving the outcomes required by NCLB and indicated by available research syntheses. We begin by recounting the four major sources of vulnerability to school violence introduced in Chapter 1, and provide the rationale for conducting a thorough assessment of each area.

FOUR SOURCES OF VULNERABILITY TO SCHOOL VIOLENCE

Defining a safe school as one without serious violence is a typical practice of school and community leaders. However, adopting such a view may lead school leaders toward narrowly focused and expensive approaches: If the only goal of school safety planning is to prevent school shootings, overuse of law enforcement and/or school security technology may be the result (Green, 1999). Although often necessary and appropriate, these approaches need to be balanced with the overall mission of schooling, which is to promote academic excellence, socialization, citizenship, and healthy lives for our children.

Students who display antisocial or violent behavior present serious risks to the safety and climate of *any* school (Kaufman et al., 2000). However, the presence of substantial numbers of antisocial students in a school is not the *only* risk to its safety. The four major sources of vulnerability to the safety of school settings (Sprague et al., 2002) illustrate the range of influences on school safety and security: (1) the physical layout of the school building and the supervision/use of school space; (2) the administrative, teaching, and management practices of the school; (3) the characteristics of the surrounding neighborhoods served by the school; and (4) the characteristics of the students enrolled in the school. This section defines and outlines each source of vulnerability and describes suggested measures for assessing it.

Typically, in the search for school safety solutions, educators often focus exclusively on individual student backgrounds, attitudes, and behavioral characteristics. The student is viewed as *the problem*. However, the remaining three sources of vulnerability are very significant in accounting for the safety of today's schools.

Ensuring the safety and security of students and staff members in our schools is a very complex responsibility that requires a comprehensive approach. Our society's myriad social problems (e.g., the abuse and neglect of children, societal fragmentation, rage, increasing incidence of interpersonal violence) are spilling over into schools at an alarming rate, and yet we have a poor understanding of how each of these factors contributes to school safety. It is essential that school leaders assess and address each of these four areas systematically in order to create safe and effective school environs. With proper and thorough assessment, teams of school personnel, parents, and others can identify, plan for, and reduce the risk factors that move schools in the direction of violence and reduced safety.

The Physical Layout of the School Building and Grounds

Perhaps the most neglected of the four sources of vulnerability is the architectural design of the school building and surrounding grounds (Schneider et al., 2000; DeMary, Owens, & Ramnarain, 2000). School safety and security were not dominant concerns when most of our school facilities were designed. School planners have paid relatively less attention to this area in the past, perhaps because school safety was not a pressing issue and ranked lower on the list of considerations that drive school design. However, the knowledge base required for designing safer schools has existed for years. This knowledge base, relating to the influence of the social and physical environment on safety and security, has emerged over the past four decades (Schneider et al., 2000), and it has been organized and formulated into a set of principles known as Crime Prevention through Environmental Design (CPTED). CPTED helps us to understand how the physical environment affects human behavior. It can be used to improve the management and use of physical spaces in both school and nonschool settings. CPTED has been used extensively in the prevention and deterrence of criminal behavior in a range of community settings. CPTED also has been applied with considerable effectiveness in making school sites safer and more secure in recent years (Schneider et al., 2000).

Weaknesses in the overall architectural design of the school can be difficult or expensive to overcome through retrofitting in older buildings. Reasonable security arrangements can reduce, but not totally eliminate, the absolute risk of an armed intruder or other violent incidents (Schneider et al., 2000; Fein et al., 2002). Recommended arrangements in this context include the following:

1. *Closed campus*. Closing school campuses during school hours simplifies surveillance demands and helps prevent entry by unauthorized persons.
2. *Security cameras*. Strategically placed cameras can be deterrents by themselves and may assist in identifying intruders.
3. *Staff and visitor identification badges*. Visitors, staff, and substitutes should be asked to check in at the office and wear identifying badges.
4. *Volunteer or campus supervisors*. Volunteers can assist with building supervision before school and during lunch, patrolling school grounds and talking to students. Teachers or school resource officers can each be assigned a period throughout the day to walk around and monitor activity on campus.
5. *Two-way communication systems*. All adults in the school should have the ability to achieve two-way communication with the front office at all times, without leaving the classroom or otherwise entering a dangerous situation.
6. *Child study teams*. Building administrators, school psychologists, counselors, and others should meet together regularly to review the adjustment status of students in the school, especially those who have generated concerns in any staff member or parent. In this context, problem solving takes place and action plans are developed that range from continued monitoring to intervention.
7. *Lockdown procedure*. Building emergency procedures should be reviewed with staff each fall, included in the staff handbook, and practiced by all staff and students, much like the traditional fire drill.
8. *Confidential reporting system*. The school should make available to students, parents, and staff a confidential reporting system through which potential "incidents," to occur during school or non-school hours, can be revealed. Options include anonymous "tip lines" or web-based applications, such as *www.report-it.com*.
9. *School resource officers*. Schools increasingly use either sworn public safety officers or community safety personnel to supervise students, provide training, and intervene in conflicts or illegal activity.

In the wake of recent, highly publicized school shootings, some have advocated a high-security architectural design for schools using metal detectors, locked gates, video surveillance cameras, etc. However, a well-designed school should look like a place to learn—not a locked-down fortress (Green, 1999). Prudent application of CPTED principles of security technology can satisfy both perspectives. Architectural features that allow natural surveillance *and* provide controlled access to the school create an environment that can reduce risk of violence while enhancing, rather than detracting from, the learning climate.

The Administrative, Teaching, and Management Practices of the School

Schools have been identified as the ideal setting for organizing efforts against the increasing problems of children and youth who display antisocial behavior (Mayer, 1995; Sugai & Horner, 1994; Walker et al., 1996). Effective interventions must be implemented that (1) apply a multiple-systems approach to schoolwide discipline aimed at *all* students, (2) support educators in today's classrooms and schools, and (3) adopt and sustain evidence-based, cost-efficient practices that actually work as intended (Gottfredson, 1997; 2001; Walker et al., 1996). Effective approaches to schoolwide discipline and management, for example, include (1) systematic social skills instruction in key areas (e.g., conflict resolution education, drug and alcohol resistance curriculum, etc.), (2) academic or curricular restructuring, (3) positive, behaviorally based interventions, (4) early screening and identification of antisocial behavior patterns, and (5) alternatives to traditional suspension and expulsion (Biglan, 1995; Lipsey, 1991; Mayer, 1995; Sprague, Sugai, & Walker, 1998; Sugai & Horner, 1994; Tobin & Sprague, 2000; Tolan & Guerra, 1994; Walker, Colvin, & Ramsey, 1995; Walker et al., 1996).

We recommend that program selection be based on a thorough assessment of school discipline practices (Sugai et al., 2000), disciplinary referral patterns (Sugai, Sprague, Horner & Walker, 2000), academic instruction, and whole-school social skills teaching. As noted above, thorough needs assessments can guide planning, avoid overlapping or conflicting services, and serve as the basis for evaluation of change. In addition, accomplishing high-magnitude change in schools requires an appropriate and sustained investment in staff development and provision of data-based feedback to school personnel (Hawkins, Catalano, Kosterman, Abbott, & Hill, 1999; Sprague, Walker, Golly, et al., 2001).

In Chapter 1 we introduced School-Wide Positive Behavior Support (SWPBS), which is a system of providing training, technical assistance, and evaluation of school discipline and climate. SWPBS is a multisystemic, whole-school approach to addressing the special problems posed by antisocial students and coping with challenging forms of student behavior, in general.

The key practices of SWPBS include (1) clear definitions of expected appropriate, positive behaviors; (2) clear definitions of problem behaviors and their consequences; (3) regularly scheduled instruction and assistance in desired positive social behaviors; (4) effective incentives and motivational systems; (5) school staff committed to staying with the intervention over the long term; (6) staff who receive training, feedback, and coaching about effective implementation of the intervention; and (7) established systems for measuring and monitoring the intervention's effectiveness. These practices can greatly decrease office discipline problems and increase consistency of communication among adults in the school. Chapter 3 describes a comprehensive staff development curriculum designed to achieve implementation of SWPBS practices.

Characteristics of Surrounding Neighborhoods

The contexts in which school-influencing risk factors exist include the family, neighborhood, community, and the larger society (Hawkins & Catalano, 1992). Across these contexts, contributing risk factors can include poverty, dysfunctional and chaotic family life, drug and alcohol abuse by primary caregivers, domestic abuse, neglect, emotional and physical abuse, negative attitudes toward schooling, the modeling of physical intimidation and aggression, sexual exploitation, excessive exposure to media violence, the growing incivility of our society, and so on. These risk factors nurture the development of antisocial attitudes and coercive behavioral styles in the children who are pervasively exposed to them.

Assessment of neighborhood and family characteristics can be accomplished, in large measure, by using archival data collected (often routinely) by law enforcement, child protective services, juvenile authorities, and health departments. We illustrate the constructive use of these information sources later in this chapter.

Characteristics of the Students Enrolled in the School

Our schools are made unsafe by the attitudes, beliefs, and dangerous behavior patterns of antisocial children and youth who attend them. These characteristics are stimulated by the risk factors listed above regarding family, community, and society. The task of schools, families, and communities is to promote resilience, teach skills for school success, and develop positive alternatives to replace the maladaptive forms of behavior the at-risk or delinquent/antisocial child has learned to use in achieving his or her social goals.

In any school, we would expect to find three relatively distinct populations of students: (1) typically developing students, (2) those at-risk for behavioral and academic problems, and (3) high-risk students who already manifest serious behavioral and academic difficulties (Sprague & Walker, 2000). Differing but complementary approaches are necessary to address the needs of these three student groups. Figure 2.1 illustrates the typical distribution of students of each type and indicates the level of intervention each needs. Assessing and identifying the characteristics of students in a school includes identifying rates of juvenile arrests or contacts with law enforcement, the frequency and severity of discipline referrals in school, the proportion of students living in poverty, academic achievement levels, social skills development, and so forth.

As seen above, the characterization of a school as safe or unsafe is a complex task involving assessment of several interrelated dimensions. In the remainder of this chapter we outline procedures for conducting essential needs assessment and intervention selection activities. This section uses the organizational framework of the four sources of vulnerability.

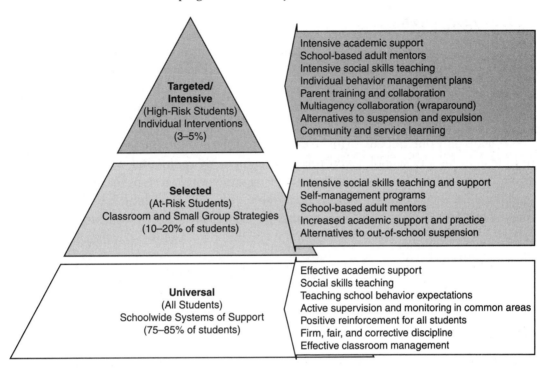

FIGURE 2.1. Three-tiered model of schoolwide discipline strategies.

THE "HOW TO" OF SCHOOL SAFETY PLANNING AND INTERVENTION

We recommend use of the United States Department of Education (USDOE) Office of Safe and Drug Free Schools' "Principles of Effectiveness" as an organizing framework for planning and implementing schoolwide safety approaches, as outlined at the beginning of this chapter. These steps include (1) conducting a local needs assessment of the risk and protective factors affecting school sites; (2) establishment of measurable goals and objectives by the school in collaboration with families; and (3) selection of research-based and research-validated curricula and interventions: In this section we discuss each step and provide example applications.

Conducting a Local Needs Assessment

Table 2.1 provides a summary of the assessment tools we recommend for a comprehensive needs assessment. In the following material, we outline procedures for assessing risk relative to each of the four sources of vulnerability.

CPTED Assessment

Every school can benefit from an assessment of its environmental design that evaluates features pertaining to whether the school is a safe and secure place to learn and work. A school site that is riddled with criminal activity has an obvious need for such an assessment, but even campuses that seem to be orderly and secure at first glance may present a multitude of risks when inspected.

It takes only one tragedy to make the benefits of preventive assessment crystal clear in hindsight for any school. Even relatively minor environmental flaws are worthy of attention and action. For example, if someone trips over broken steps because of deferred maintenance, and is injured, serious litigation may result. If nothing is done to actively discourage drug dealers or other criminals from entering school campuses, the district incurs a risk of liability that may threaten its insurability. A child who threatens violent behavior obviously cannot be ignored—which is why a risk-assessment protocol must be in place in every school (U.S. Department of Education, 2003; Fein et al., 2002). Whenever there is a history of trouble or the likelihood of future problems, eventual personal injuries, as well as subsequent legal actions, are also likely.

TABLE 2.1. Four Sources of Vulnerability to School Safety: Needs Assessment Tools

Architecture and supervision of the school building	Administrative and management practices of the school	Characteristics of the community and its families	Characteristics of students enrolled in the school
CPTED school "walk-through" assessment (Schneider et al., 2000) Oregon School Safety Survey (Sprague et al., 1995)	• Whole-school discipline practices survey • School-Wide Evaluation Tool (SET) (Sugai et al., 1999) • Faculty characteristics • Office discipline referrals (frequency, type) • Suspensions and expulsions (frequency, type)	• Poverty (free and reduced lunch status of students) • Mobility • Child abuse or domestic violence rates • Community crime rates • Community focus group information (needs, goals, barriers) • School Crime Assessment Tool (Stephens, 1995)	• School enrollment (school size) • School demographics • Academic achievement test scores • Attendance • Juvenile crime rates • Universal screening (see Chapter 6) • Alcohol, tobacco, and other drug use survey results (e.g., Effective Behavior Survey)

CPTED assessment procedures can be relatively straightforward (see Crowe, 1991; Schneider et al., 2000). The assessment process should begin with tools such as the National School Safety Center's School Crime Assessment Tool (Stephens, 1995; see Chapter 1) or the Oregon School Safety Survey (Sprague, Colvin, & Irvin, 1995; described later in this chapter and included in Form 1.2 in Chapter 1). These tools allow stakeholders to provide input on particular areas of concern to them. Following this initial assessment, a CPTED expert (local law enforcement or security personnel) is typically employed to conduct a walk-through of the school site and provide an intensive assessment. Form 2.1 at the end of the chapter provides an example of such a walk-through assessment.

Once the initial assessments of the school's relative safety have been completed, using the self-report measures described in the preceding paragraphs, the CPTED evaluation process can begin.

Conducting the School Site Evaluation

Evaluation of the school site begins with a close look at the neighborhood. Typically, neighborhood and community problems spill over directly into the school setting. Conditions noted during evaluation of the community or neighborhood will give school officials helpful clues, as they seek to devise remedies geared toward making both the school and the neighborhood safer for their students. If the surrounding neighborhood is relatively impoverished or chaotic, there is a greater likelihood that the school will experience a high level of social disorder (Gottfredson & Gottfredson, 1985). The presence of such problems indicates that student safety, en route to and from school, needs to be addressed.

Begin the CPTED assessment process by working slowly around the outside of the school while taking notes, starting away from the site and circling back in to it. An evaluation team may include an administrator, a teacher, a student, a custodian, and/or a school resource officer. Diverse team membership can bring a broad perspective and valuable information to this process. Once the walk-through is completed, more extensive planning and recommendations are formulated by a CPTED expert (e.g., a local architect or police personnel).

Conducting the School Climate Assessment

We recommend the use of three related assessment tools to evaluate the quality of positive school discipline practices and to elicit staff, parent, or community member perceptions of risk and protective factors affecting school safety: (1) the Best Behavior School Discipline Assessment, (2) the School-Wide Evaluation Tool (Sugai, Lewis-Palmer, Todd, & Horner, 1999), and (3) the Oregon School Safety Survey. Each is described here, using sample data summaries and decision rules to illustrate recommended use.

Each year the school's positive behavior support team, or the entire staff, should be asked to voluntarily rate the status of several features of research validated school discipline practices, using the Best Behavior School Discipline Assessment (BBSDA). This checklist asks raters to indicate the extent to which a school discipline practice is in place across schools (including common areas), classrooms, and family and individual student support systems (see Chapter 3 for a full description and a copy of the survey). Sample items include questions regarding the structure and functioning of the building-based team (i.e., whether school rules, appropriate recognition and incentives, and reinforcement systems are in place, etc.) We recommend using the assessment annually to ascertain the quality of intervention implementation from the perspective of staff participating in the intervention. Those items that are rated as "not in place" should be targeted for improvement by the SWPBS team.

The School-Wide Evaluation Tool (SET; Sugai et al., 1999) was developed to measure whether, and how well, school personnel are implementing the practices and systems associated with schoolwide positive behavior support. Data to complete the 28 items of the SET are collected by an on-site observer, who reviews school documents, examines physical spaces, interviews staff, and interviews students over a 60–90-minute period. Each SET item is scored as "in place," "partially in place," or "not in place." The SET produces a summary score (0–100%) and seven subscale scores: (1) schoolwide behavioral expectations are defined; (2) expectations are taught; (3) rewards are provided for following the behavioral expectations; (4) a continuum of consequences for problem behavior is in place; (5) data on problem behavior are collected and used for decision making, (6) an administrator actively supports schoolwide PBS, and (7) the school district supports schoolwide PBS. A school meets criterion as "implementing schoolwide PBS" when the SET results indicate a summary score $\geq$ 80% and an "expectations taught" subscale score $\geq$ 80%.

Horner et al. (2004) report internal consistency reliability of the SET at an overall alpha level of .96, with a test–retest level of 97.3% (at 2 weeks). The validity of the SET was evaluated within Messick's (1988) unified construct validity framework. Summary SET scores from 31 elementary schools were compared with scores from the schoolwide section of the Effective Behavior Support Self-Assessment Survey (another recommended school discipline assessment measure; Horner et al., 2004) and produced a Pearson $r = .75$ ($p \leq .01$). Subscale scores of the SET also were demonstrated to correlate acceptably with the SET summary score (median $r = .65$; range .44–.81), indicating acceptable internal consistency.

By addressing questions within each of the seven features listed above, the information gathered from the SET can be used to (1) assess features that are in place, (2) determine annual goals for schoolwide effective behavior support, (3) evaluate ongoing efforts toward schoolwide behavior support, (4) design and revise procedures, as needed, and (5) compare efforts expended on schoolwide effective behavior support from year to year. A copy of the SET can be obtained from Anne Todd or Rob Horner at the University of

Oregon. Figure 2.2 provides sample results from a SET school assessment. This graph shows 3 years of progress for one school, across the seven subscales.

In order to assess important safety concerns, the Oregon School Safety Survey (Sprague et al., 1995; see Chapters 1 and 3) should be administered annually to all key school stakeholders (e.g., parents, teachers, administrators, classified staff, even students). The survey asks respondents to rate the presence and extent of 17 risk and 16 protective factors associated with increases or decreases in school violence and discipline problems. Risk factors include poverty, child abuse, bullying, deteriorating physical facilities, and graffiti. Protective factors include positive teacher–student relationships, parent involvement, student supervision, and high academic expectations. A Likert rating scale of 1 (not at all) to 4 (extensive) is used to produce average ratings for each item.

Table 2.2 provides a comparison of the top-five-rated risk and protective factors from two large samples of Oregon principals in 1995 and 2000. Whereas top-rated risk factors in 1995 focused primarily on issues outside the school (poverty, transiency, child abuse), the 2000 ratings focused on school bullying and deteriorating school facil-

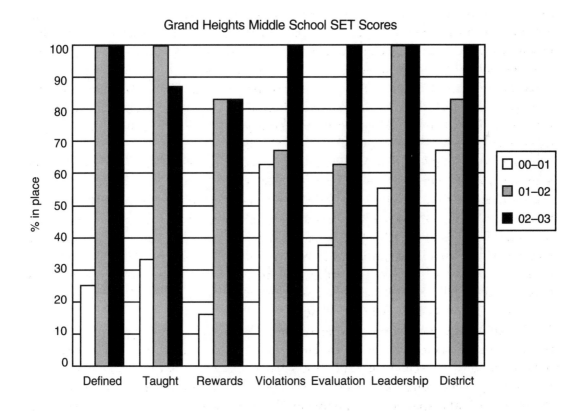

FIGURE 2.2. Sample SET school assessment results.

TABLE 2.2. Top-Rated Risk and Protective Factors from Full Sample

Top risk factors				Top protective factors			
1995	Mean	2000	Mean	1995	Mean	2000	Mean
Poverty	2.9	Bullying	3.1	Teacher–student relationships	3.6	Response to conflict	3.6
Transiency	2.9	Deteriorating facilities	3.1	Climate	3.6	Suicide prevention	3.6
Child abuse in the home	2.6	Poverty	2.9	Discipline	3.6	Staff training	3.5
Truancy	2.5	Transiency	2.8	Academic expectations	3.5	Academic expectations	3.4
Bullying	2.4	Child abuse in the home	2.4	Supervision	3.5	Parent involvement	3.4

ities, poverty, transiency, and child abuse in the home. Top-rated protective factors (indicators of what schools do best to support students) in 1995 included positive teacher–student relationships, positive school climate, school discipline, high academic expectations, and student supervision. The rankings changed dramatically in 2000 and included responses to conflict, suicide prevention programs, staff training, high academic expectations, and parent involvement. These changes likely reflect renewed emphasis on staff development as a result of academic reforms, increased funding for school discipline reform, school safety initiatives, and an emphasis on violence prevention resulting from the school shootings in Oregon and elsewhere.

Individual schools should use results from their survey for purposes of planning, decision making, goal setting, and allocation of resources. For instance, in the sample survey results, bullying and harassment in the school are rated as the number one risk factor. One decision that might be made based on this information would be to fund new or supplementary interventions aimed at decreasing bullying and harassment, or perhaps increasing funding for existing programs already in place in order to increase their efficacy, scope and reach, and chances for success.

Setting Measurable Goals and Objectives and Selecting Evidence-Based Strategies

The U.S. Public Health Service (PHS) has developed a classification system that provides for the coordinated integration of differing intervention approaches necessary to address the divergent needs of the three student types, present in different proportions in every school (i.e., not at risk, at risk, severely at risk). The three prevention approaches in the U.S. PHS classification system are primary, secondary, and tertiary. *Primary prevention* refers to the use of approaches that prevent problems from emerging; *secondary prevention* addresses those who already have problems but are not yet of a chronic nature or severe magnitude; and *tertiary prevention* uses the most powerful intervention approaches available to address the problems of severely at-risk individuals. Walker and his colleagues have outlined an integrated prevention model for schools, based on this classification system, for addressing school-based antisocial behavior patterns (Walker et al., 1996).

Universal interventions—those applied to everyone in the same manner and degree—are used to achieve primary prevention goals; that is, to keep problems from emerging. We would expect these interventions to benefit both high- and low-risk schools. Good examples of such interventions are (1) implementing a schoolwide discipline plan, (2) the schoolwide teaching of conflict resolution and violence prevention skills, (3) establishing high and consistent academic expectations for all students, and (4) providing positive reinforcement for rule following. Many of the chapters in this book provide detailed descriptions of how these important interventions can be implemented to improve school climate.

Individualized interventions applied to one case at a time or to small groups of at-risk individuals (e.g., alternative classrooms or "schools within schools") are used to achieve secondary and tertiary prevention goals. Typically, these interventions are labor intensive, complex, intrusive, and often costly, but they can be very powerful if properly implemented. They are necessary to address the more severe problems of chronically at-risk students who "select" themselves by not responding to primary prevention approaches and by demonstrating a need for much more intensive intervention services and supports. Often, implementation of these interventions is preceded by a functional behavior assessment process (Crone & Horner, 2003; O'Neill et al., 1997) to identify the conditions (e.g., antecedents and consequences) that sustain and motivate the problem behavior. We also recommend a comprehensive assessment of family, school, and individual *risk* (e.g., Achenbach, 1991; Walker & McConnell, 1995b; Walker & Severson, 1990) and *protective* factors (Epstein & Sharma, 1998) to guide delivery of broader ecological interventions.

Although this integrated model has rarely been implemented fully in the context of schooling, it nonetheless provides an ideal means for schools to develop, implement, and monitor a comprehensive management system that addresses the needs of *all* students. It is also a fair system, in that typically developing students are not penalized by being denied access to potentially beneficial interventions. In addition, it has the potential to positively impact the operations, administration, and overall climate of the school. Through its emphasis on the use of primary prevention goals, achieved through universal interventions, this model maximizes the efficient use of school resources and provides a supportive context for the application of necessary secondary and tertiary interventions for the more severely involved students. Finally, it provides a built-in screening and assessment process; that is, through careful monitoring of students' responses to the primary prevention interventions, it is possible to detect, through their unresponsiveness, those who are at greater risk and in need of more intensive services and supports.

Chapters 3 through 7 describe recommended evidence-based practices at each of the three levels. To reiterate, Chapter 1 recommended the following strategic approaches to move schools in the direction of greater safety and reduce the likelihood, over time, of a school tragedy occurring: (1) secure the school; (2) address the peer culture and its problems (see Chapter 4); (3) involve parents in making the school safer; (4) create a positive, inclusive school culture (Walker, Sprague, & Severson, 2004; see Chapter 3); and (5) develop a written school safety and crisis-response plan. We describe procedures for developing a crisis-response plan here.

DEVELOPING A WRITTEN CRISIS-RESPONSE PLAN

In today's social environment, it is essential that each school go through a planning process designed to reduce the likelihood of a school tragedy and to manage a crisis if it occurs (U.S. Department of Education, 2003; Association of California School Administrators, 1995; DeMary, et al., 2002; U.S. Department of Education Office for Civil Rights and the National Association of Attorneys General, 1999). The establishment, coordination, and maintenance of the multiple critical elements needed for an effective and efficient crisis-response capacity takes time, effort, and commitment of resources at all levels. School-based crisis-planning and response programs should address policy and procedural organization at three levels: state, district, and individual school. State-level efforts should address the legal standards, rights, and responsibilities pertaining to crisis situations and crisis management at all organizational levels, and any resources and supports to be provided at the district and individual school levels. State-level efforts are typically mandated, established, and guided by legislative process and law, and implemented and enforced by each state's Department of Education (U.S. Department of Education Office for Civil Rights and the National Association of Attorneys General, 1999).

District-level organization should set overall standards for compliance with state policy and procedure and any other local policy and procedure deemed essential to the safety of the school and community. Although it is advisable that a state-level crisis team or organization be established, it is essential to establish and maintain a district-level crisis team. The district-level crisis team responsibilities should include (1) overseeing and coordinating school-level crisis teams, (2) authorizing or providing resources when necessary, (3) disseminating information to community stakeholders, (4) providing for ongoing school-level training and educational materials, (5) monitoring and evaluating before-and-after-event crisis planning and procedures, (6) overseeing follow-up and closure activities, and (7) collaborating with community support agencies (DeMary et al., 2002; Fein et al., 2002).

It is at the individual school level that the "rubber meets the road." School-based crisis activities need to be supported and directed by a team or organizational unit that includes the administrator(s); administrative staff member(s); school-based specialists (e.g., nurse/medical staff, school resource officer, transportation and maintenance/custodial personnel); both classified and certified staff members; parents and other community stakeholders; and, when appropriate, students. There should be a clear leadership presence guiding the team's efforts—typically the principal or other administrator—and all team members should be drawn from personnel that are on campus full time (thereby increasing the likelihood that they will be present if a crisis event occurs; Paine & Sprague, 2002).

Key to any effort in crisis planning and response is the establishment of policies and procedures to guide and direct efforts in the event of a crisis. Policy and procedure are important for these reasons:

1. Establish crisis management organization.
2. Define what constitutes a crisis.
3. Define roles and responsibilities.
4. Define crisis activities and procedures.
5. Establish response protocols.
6. Provide for the dissemination of information and establish organization and coordination of various community and agency efforts.
7. Provide for the education and training of crisis-response personnel.

Simply put, people need to know what they should do, what their role might be, and who will do what, in the event of a school crisis—before, during, and after an emergency. In addition, people involved or otherwise affected need to know where to go for information and access to services—before, during, and after a crisis. Additionally, all school and community members who may be affected by, or involved in, a crisis situation or event need to receive training and education in crisis-response procedures. To paraphrase Ron Stephens, Executive Director of the National School Safety Center, "There are those who have faced a crisis, and those who are about to."

Essential to, and in conjunction with, all activities surrounding and involved in crisis planning, management, and response is a comprehensive crisis evaluation and needs assessment procedure. This procedure should accomplish the following:

• Identify potential crises.
• Identify general response activities and procedures that are, or are not, present in the school.

- Identify various emergency and crisis-response skills and capacities present, available, or needed.
- Inventory communications and support resources and procedures.
- Identify and provide for special needs populations and situations.

Form 2.2 at the end of the chapter provides a recommended school-based checklist on crisis-response procedure. When voluntarily completed by as many staff as possible, this checklist can help identify areas of strength and concern in terms of crisis planning and readiness. Furthermore, it can assist intervention planning efforts, resource allocation, and the development of the school-based crisis procedures.

CONCLUSION

An enormous amount of federal and state resources has been, and continues to be, invested in school safety and violence prevention following the school shooting tragedies of the past decade. It is extremely important that these precious resources be used to promote the adoption of best professional practices and that proven, evidence-based interventions are implemented in supporting them. These developments also create significant opportunities for school professionals (e.g., counselors, general educators, school psychologists, special educators, social workers) to collaborate more effectively and to forge new working relationships with families and community agencies.

If we could implement, with integrity, that which we currently know regarding these problems, a major positive impact would be achieved. The stakes are high for our society, our school systems, and especially our children. The potential gains are well worth the investment and effort. Careful assessment and planning for school safety form the cornerstone for any school's success.

FORM 2.1. SAMPLE SCHOOL CPTED WALK-THROUGH ASSESSMENT

Date: _____

School Name: _____

Characterize Locale and Area: Urban ____ Suburban ____ Rural ____

Industrial ____ Residential ____

Business ____ Other ____

Area	Focus	Item	Y/N	Comments
Grounds	Fences	1. Full (school grounds completely enclosed) 2. Partial (school grounds partially enclosed) 3. None	1. 2. 3.	
		1. Gated 2. Pedestrian control provided 3. Open access 4. Breached sections 5. Other	1. 2. 3. 4. 5.	
	Playgrounds	1. View of all structures/areas 2. Litter 3. Hazardous objects 4. Dangerous/broken equipment 5. ATOD (alcohol, tobacco, and other drug use)	1. 2. 3. 4. 5.	
	Parking lots, street access, pickup/dropoff	1. View of all areas 2. Litter 3. Hazardous objects 4. Vandalism 5. Signs 6. Traffic control 7. Crosswalks 8. Bus areas marked and clear 9. Visitor's parking 10. ATOD use visible	1. 2. 3. 4. 5. 6. 7. 8. 9. 10.	

(continued)

FORM 2.1. *(page 2 of 3)*

Area	Focus	Item	Y/N	Comments
Building	Outside	1. Vandalism 2. Graffiti 3. Broken windows 4. Broken doors 5. General infrastructure 6. ATOD 7. Signs (no trespassing, no dogs, etc.)	1. 2. 3. 4. 5. 6. 7.	
	A. Lines of sight	1. Bushes 2. Trees 3. Outbuildings 4. Hidden/obscured areas	1. 2. 3. 4.	
	B. Access and visitor control	1. Doors locked/secured 2. Direction signs to entrance 3. Intruder alarms and alert protocols 4. Video surveillance	1. 2. 3. 4.	
	Inside			
	A. Access and visitor control	1. View of entrance from office 2. Entry/exit control 3. Rules, regulations, expectations posted 4. Sign in/sign out 5. Visible visitor and staff ID 6. Video surveillance	1. 2. 3. 4. 5. 6.	
	B. Student	1. Random locker checks 2. Visible student ID (high and middle schools) 3. Student access to reporting protocols (hotlines, anonymous reports, clearly identified responsible staff, etc.) 4. Process taught to students and staff at least twice a year	1. 2. 3. 4.	

(continued)

Crisis	A. School community	1. Written policy and process for responding to fighting or other violence	1.	
		2. Staff members trained to safely and effectively intervene in student violence	2.	
		3. Written policy and process for reporting crime (student and staff)	3.	
		4. School response processes for various emergency situations (earthquake, fire, etc.) are established and disseminated throughout the school community	4.	
		5. Policies and processes are taught to students and staff at least twice a year	5.	
		6. School access to, and coordination with, local law enforcement and other community emergency service providers is established	6.	
	B. Building	1. Sprinklers, fire extinguishers, etc., are present, inspected, and in working order	1.	
		2. Emergency medical equipment is provided, inspected, and in working order	2.	
		3. Emergency exits are clearly marked and accessible	3.	
		4. Physical access to school by community emergency personnel and equipment is clearly marked and accessible	4.	
Comments				

FORM 2.2. CRISIS PLANNING AND RESPONSE CHECKLIST

School: _____   Date: _____

Check the crisis response plan or procedures that are present in your school:

- ❏ Tornado
- ❏ Fire
- ❏ Hurricane
- ❏ Earthquake
- ❏ Armed intruder
- ❏ Unarmed intruder
- ❏ Bomb threat/explosion
- ❏ Hazmat exposure
- ❏ Threats to school/students (phone, letter, message, etc.)
- ❏ Serious fight
- ❏ Accidental death or serious injury
- ❏ Other natural disaster
- ❏ Air or train disaster (if applicable)
- ❏ Emergency evacuation
- ❏ Emergency utility shutoff
- ❏ Other _____

	Yes	No
1. The school has a crisis-response team (either district- or site-based).	❏	❏
2. All staff and all students are trained in crisis-response procedures at least once a year.	❏	❏
3. Drills are conducted on all crisis-response procedures at least twice a year.	❏	❏
4. Each staff member is assigned a primary crisis responsibility.	❏	❏
5. Classrooms and other rooms have doors that can lock from the inside (lockdown procedure).	❏	❏
6. Classrooms and other rooms have intercom phones or two-way radios.	❏	❏
7. The school has a clear, written procedure for reporting crime.	❏	❏
8. Outside access is controlled and entry limited.	❏	❏
9. Doors and windows are not blocked for emergency exit.	❏	❏

(continued)

	Yes	No
10. The school has clear, written procedures and established methods for visitor monitoring and control.	❏	❏
11. The school has a student search policy and procedures in place.	❏	❏
12. The school has a computer use and crime policy in place.	❏	❏
13. The school has an anti-harassment/anti-bullying policy and procedure in place.	❏	❏
14. The school has anti-gang policies and procedures in place.	❏	❏
15. The school conducts a student safety survey at least annually.	❏	❏
16. The school conducts a teacher and staff safety survey at least annually.	❏	❏
17. School discipline plans and policies are provided to all school community members (students, staff, parents, etc.) at least once a year.	❏	❏
18. School behavior expectations and discipline plans and policies are taught to, and reviewed with, all students at least twice a year.	❏	❏
19. The school conducts a risk/threat assessment a least once a year.	❏	❏
20. The school conducts a CPTED (Crime Prevention through Environmental Design) assessment at least once a year.	❏	❏

Does the school have:

❏ Clearly written behavior expectations
❏ Behavior expectations disseminated to parents, students, and staff
❏ Expectations posted in all school areas
❏ A schoolwide discipline plan
❏ A discipline referral database
❏ A clear method of contacting emergency medical services
❏ A clear method of contacting local law enforcement
❏ A clear method of contacting other community emergency services (fire, etc.)
❏ A procedure for reporting crime
❏ A policy for communicating with families in the event of a crisis
❏ A protocol for student risk/threat assessment

3

Improving School Climate, Safety, and Student Health with Schoolwide Positive Behavior Supports

Hoping to prevent minor discipline problems as well as more serious antisocial and violent incidents, many schools have turned to a schoolwide positive discipline approach, commonly referred to as School-Wide Positive Behavior Support (SWPBS; Osher, Dwyer, & Jackson, 2003; Sugai, Horner, & Gresham, 2002; Sprague & Golly, 2004), as a foundation response. SWPBS is based on the assumption that when all school staff members within in all school settings actively teach and consistently recognize and reinforce appropriate behavior, the number of students with serious behavior problems will be reduced and the school's overall climate will improve (Colvin, Kame'enui, & Sugai, 1993; Sugai & Lewis, 1999; Sugai & Horner, 2002; Sugai, Lewis-Palmer, Todd, & Horner, 2000).

SWPBS schools aim to (1) create a positive school climate, (2) establish and teach behavioral expectations schoolwide, and (3) teach mastery and encourage demonstration of behavioral skills (e.g., compliance to school rules, safe and respectful peer-to-peer interactions, academic effort/engagement) that will alter the trajectory of at-risk children toward destructive outcomes and prevent the onset of risk behavior in typically developing children. Its effective and sustained implementation is likely to create a more responsive school climate that supports the twin goals of schooling for all children: *academic achievement* and *social development* (Walker, Irvin, & Sprague, 1997).

Having an organized, schoolwide system in place for behavior management and social skills training is the foundation of effective prevention. In addition to the direct benefit such a system has on student behavior in school, it creates the context for school-based efforts to support effective parenting. When school personnel share a vision of the kind of social behavior they want to promote among students and an understanding of the type of social environment that is needed to achieve such behavior, they are in a position to inform and reinforce families in their efforts to create the same kind of supportive environment at home. When educators are clear about how to use rules, positive reinforcement, and consistent, mildly negative consequences to support behavioral development, they are better able to coordinate their efforts with those of parents. As a result, parents know more about their children's behavior in school and are able to provide the same supports and consequences that the school is providing.

This chapter describes how to establish and implement a schoolwide, positive discipline plan that includes needs assessment, implementation, and evaluation phases. A highly acclaimed staff development program called *Best Behavior* (Sprague & Golly, 2004) is showcased as an exemplary approach in this regard. We begin by outlining the scope of today's school discipline problem and its relationship to school safety.

THE CHALLENGE OF SCHOOL DISCIPLINE

Most schools in the United States are relatively safe places for children, youth, and the adults who teach and support them (U.S. Departments of Justice and Education, 1999, 2000). However, fears about the personal safety of students, teachers, parents, and community members are very real and need to be addressed. It also is true that some schools have serious crime and violence problems and that most schools are having to deal with more serious problem behaviors (e.g., bullying, harassment, victimization, drug and alcohol abuse, the effects of family disruption, poverty; Kingery, 1999).

No school is immune to challenging behaviors. Such behaviors exist in every school and community, and they always will. The extent of the challenge varies in intensity and frequency across schools, and, as noted previously, the onset and development of antisocial behavior are associated with a variety of school, community, and family risk factors (Sprague et al., 2002; Walker & Sylwester, 1991; see Chapter 2 for a description of student, family, and neighborhood risk factors, and Chapter 5 for a description of the major individual risk factors). Our challenge is to reduce the frequency and intensity of these problems and to sustain our success over time.

The social problems noted above compete directly with the instructional mission of schools. The result is decreased academic achievement and a lower quality of life for students and staff alike. The *National Educational Goals Panel Report* (U.S. Department of Education, 1998) lists five essential areas in which national school performance has declined: (1) reading achievement at Grade 12 has decreased (Goal 3); (2)

student drug use has increased (Goal 7); (3) sale of drugs at school in grades 8, 10, and 12 has increased; (4) threats and injuries to public school teachers have increased (Goal 7); and, (5) more teachers are reporting that disruptions in their classroom interfere with their teaching (Goal 7). These undesirable outcomes illustrate the clear link between school climate, school violence, and academic achievement. We cannot achieve national educational goals and meaningful reform without addressing these disturbing conditions (Elias, Zins, Graczyk, & Weissberg, 2004).

SCHOOL PRACTICES CONTRIBUTING TO THE PROBLEM

Many school practices contribute to the development of antisocial behavior and the potential for violence. Because of an overemphasis on detecting individual child or youth characteristics that predict violence or disruption, as noted previously, many important systemic variables are often overlooked (Colvin et al., 1993; Hawkins, Catalano, Kosterman, Abbott, & Hill, 1999; Mayer, 1995; Walker & Eaton-Walker, 2000; Walker et al., 1996). These include, among others:

1. Ineffective instruction that results in academic failure.
2. Inconsistent and punitive classroom and behavior-management practices.
3. Lack of opportunity to learn and practice prosocial interpersonal and self-management skills.
4. Unclear rules and expectations regarding appropriate behavior.
5. Failure to effectively correct rule violations and reward adherence to them.
6. Failure to individualize instruction and support to accommodate individual differences (e.g., ethnic and cultural differences, gender, disability).
7. Failure to assist students from at-risk backgrounds (e.g., poverty, racial/ethnic minority members) to bond with the schooling process.
8. Disagreement about, and inconsistency in, implementation among staff members.
9. Lack of administrator involvement, leadership, and support.

Common Response to Behavioral Problems: Turn to Office Referrals, Suspensions, and Expulsions

We commonly observe that when a student misbehaves, the first line of response involves increased monitoring and supervision, restating rules, and delivering sanctions such as referrals to the office, out-of-school suspension, and/or loss of privileges. The administrator may come to a point of frustration and attempt to establish a "bottom line" for disruptive students (usually, referral or suspension). Unfortunately, these "tough" responses produce immediate but short-lived relief for the school and do not facilitate the progress of the at-risk student, who may already be disengaged from the schooling process.

Although punishment practices may appear to "work" in the short term, more often than not they merely remove the student for a period of time, thus providing respite for school personnel and sometimes students. All too often, these practices also lead some to assign exclusive responsibility for effecting positive change in the troubled student to the student or family and thereby prevent meaningful school engagement and development of solutions. The use of sanctions without an accompanying program of teaching, and according recognition for, expected positive behavior may merely displace the problem elsewhere (likely, to the home or the community). There is little evidence of the long-term effect of these practices in reducing antisocial behavior (Skiba, Peterson, & Williams, 1997; Irvin, Tobin, Sprague, Sugai, & Vincent, 2004). In fact, evidence suggests that schools using punishment practices alone promote more antisocial behavior than those with a firm but fair discipline system (Mayer, 1995; Skiba et al., 1997). Research shows clearly that schools using only punishment techniques tend to have increased rates of vandalism, aggression, truancy, and school dropout (Mayer, 1995).

For students who demonstrate chronic problem behaviors, these negative practices are more likely to impair child–adult relationships and attachment to schooling than to reduce the likelihood of those problem behaviors. Punishment alone, without a balance of support and efforts to restore school engagement, weakens academic outcomes and maintains the antisocial trajectory of at-risk students. Instead, the discipline process should (1) help students accept responsibility, (2) place high value on academic engagement and achievement, (3) teach alternative ways to behave, and (4) focus on restoring a positive environment and civil social relationships in the school.

For many of us, it is difficult to admit that our own practices and behavior may actually contribute to the problem. Take a moment to reflect on the questions in Box 3.1 and consider which practices exist in your school that may be making the problems worse, or better.

If Not Punishment, Then What Is the Solution?

We believe that schools can serve as an ideal setting in which to organize efforts that address the increasing problems of children and youth who display antisocial behavior

---

BOX 3.1. Reflection

- Which practices or conditions in my school may worsen the behavior problems of students?
- Does the discipline process in my school help students to shift their focus to restoring academic achievement and cultivating positive social relationships?

patterns (Mayer, 1995; Sugai & Horner, 1994; Walker et al., 1996). This practice is sustained by a tendency to try to eliminate the presenting problem quickly (i.e., remove the student via suspension or expulsion, or fix a "within-child" deficit) rather than focusing on the administrative, teaching, and management practices that either contribute to, or reduce, them (Tobin, Sugai, & Martin, 2000).

A solid research base exists to guide a careful analysis of the administrative, teaching, and management practices in a school and construct alternatives to ineffective approaches. In any school, there are typically developing students, who engage in few problematic behaviors, and other students who engage in multiple, comorbid, and destructive patterns of perpetration and victimization of others. This requires that *interventions be implemented that target both schoolwide and individual levels.* Educators in today's schools and classrooms must be supported to adopt and sustain effective, cost-efficient practices in this regard (Gottfredson, 1997; Gottfredson, Gottfredson, & Czeh, 2000; Walker et al., 1996).

Changing School Climate Is an Essential Element

The biggest challenge we face is to enhance our overall capacity to create and sustain positive and effective schools. We should begin schoolwide prevention activities early, keep at it, and never quit (O'Donnell, Hawkins, Catalano, Abbott, & Day, 1995). We know it is never too late or never too early to support children and youth in our schools (Loeber & Farrington, 1998b). Research indicates that schools can foster resilient, engaged students, provide students with valued roles and meaningful responsibilities, and establish clear expectations for learning and positive behavior while providing firm but fair discipline (Bryk & Discroll, 1988). Students are more motivated when they feel listened to; they learn skills that can be applied for years to come (Katz, 1997). Effective schools have shared values regarding mission and purpose, carry out multiple activities designed to promote prosocial behavior and connection to school traditions, and provide a caring, nurturing social climate involving collegial relationships among adults and students (Bryk & Driscoll, 1988).

A well-developed body of research evidence on school safety indicates that (1) early identification of, and intervention with, at-risk children in schools is feasible; (2) the risk of dropping out of school, delinquency, violence, and other adjustment problems is high unless these children are helped; (3) academic recovery is difficult if early intervention is not provided; and (4) universal interventions need to be combined with interventions targeted to specific problems (Gottfredson, 2001; Tolan, Gorman-Smith, & Henry, 2001).

Our challenge becomes how to give schools the capacity to adopt and sustain the processes, organizational structures, and systems that would enable them to carry out these effective interventions (Gottfredson et al., 2000). The problem for schools is not the lack of *effective* programs (i.e., those that work) but one of *efficacy* (i.e., helping typical schools adopt and carry out effective interventions).

SCHOOLWIDE, POSITIVE DISCIPLINE: HOW TO GET THERE

As introduced in Chapters 1 and 2, SWPBS is a systems-based approach that promotes safe and orderly schools. Researchers at the University of Oregon (see Sprague, Sugai, & Walker, 1998; Sprague, Walker, Golly, et al., 2001; Sugai & Horner, 1994; Taylor-Greene et al., 1997; *www.pbis.org*) have extensively field-tested and researched the efficacy of SWPBS approaches in reducing school behavior problems and promoting a positive school climate. As noted in Chapter 2, SWPBS is a multisystemic approach to addressing the problems posed by antisocial students and to coping with challenging forms of student behavior. The key practices of SWPBS include the following elements:

1. Clear definitions of expected behaviors (i.e., appropriate, positive) are provided to students and staff members.
2. Clear definitions of problem behaviors and their consequences are defined for students and staff members.
3. Regularly scheduled instruction *and* assistance regarding desired positive social behaviors is provided to enable students to acquire the necessary skills to effect the needed behavior changes.
4. Effective incentives and motivational systems are provided that encourage students to behave differently.
5. Staff commit to implementing the intervention over the long term and to monitoring, supporting, coaching, debriefing, and providing booster lessons for students, as necessary, to maintain the achieved gains.
6. Staff receive training, feedback, and coaching in the effective implementation of the systems.
7. Systems for measuring and monitoring the intervention's effectiveness are established.

Improvement of Discipline

First, we recommend that improvement of school discipline be one of the top school goals. Given the reality of competing resources and goals, progress will be difficult if work in this area is not prioritized.

Commitment of Administrator

Every school needs a principal who is committed to SWPBS leadership and participation. In the absence of administrative leadership and district support (e.g., policy, fiscal impediments), it will be difficult to effect broad-based changes. Hallinger and Heck (1998) reviewed the evidence of a principal's contribution to a school's effectiveness in providing SWPBS. They concluded that principals exercise a measurable effect on schooling effectiveness and student achievement. Kam, Greenberg, and Walls (2003) reported that the ability of principals to initiate and sustain innovations in their schools is related to successful program implementation. The length of time administrators have spent in the school setting and the leadership characteristics they show in maintaining good relations with teachers, parents, school boards, site councils, and students also are positively related to successful implementation outcomes. Gottfredson et al. (2000) and Ingersoll (2001) showed that high levels of administrative support were also associated with reduced staff turnover.

Commitment of Staff

We have found it important to secure a commitment to implement the intervention by at least 80% of school staff. Some schools have chosen to use a "vote" to assess this level of commitment. We have found the following approaches useful in moving your colleagues toward program implementation (Embry, 2004).

• *Talk about cost and benefit.* All adults involved need to know the costs (i.e., time, funds) and benefits of working to improve school discipline. Presentations by school leaders on the anticipated effects of program adoption (e.g., our experience indicates that discipline problems are dramatically reduced, as are referrals to the principal's office, and teaching time is substantially increased) are especially helpful in this regard.

• *Emphasize the long-term benefits.* It also is useful to discuss the "higher good" of prevention and how much everyone values such outcomes as better academic achievement, prevention of alcohol, tobacco, and other drug use, less teacher stress, etc. These discussions may prove to be more powerful and persuasive than simply appealing to authority or law (i.e., "We *have* to do it!").

• *"Try before you buy."* SWPBS is comprised of many smaller techniques (e.g., reward systems, teaching rules; Embry, 2004) that can be promoted as trial products. Innovators can be asked to share their successes or arrange visits to schools that have already adopted SWPBS practices.

• *"Go with the goers."* The practice is far more likely to be adopted if you recognize and support people who get on-board early, as well as encourage those who are reluctant or even resistant.

To begin your journey toward establishing a more effective school program, we recommend that you begin by completing the needs assessment presented in Form 3.1 at the end of the chapter (Sprague & Golly, 2004). Another excellent self-assessment is the Assessing Behavior Support in Schools survey developed by George Sugai and his colleagues (Sugai et al., 2000; available at *www.pbis.org*). We strongly recommend that all adults in the school complete this type of assessment; furthermore, you can reflect on your own views about your school's status on each item. The survey asks you to reflect on whether the practice is in place in your school and to choose which items are priorities for improvement. Once you have identified areas needing improvement, use the goals table at the end of the form to identify the goals you envision and set concrete action steps toward their attainment. Your school behavior team will refer to these goals often and modify them, as indicated, by your review of the key data you will gather regarding effectiveness (e.g., office discipline referrals, rates of problem behavior on the playground).

Selection of Evidence-Based Practices

Best Behavior (Sprague & Golly, 2004) provides a standardized staff development program aimed at improving school and classroom discipline and associated outcomes (e.g., reduction in incidence of school violence and alcohol, tobacco, and other drug use). Based on SWPBS (Sugai & Horner, 1994; Sprague et al., 1998), Best Behavior was developed at the University of Oregon and the National Center on Positive Behavioral Interventions and Supports (*www.pbis.org*; an Office of Special Education Programs funded research center). The goal of the Best Behavior program is to facilitate the academic achievement and healthy social development of children and youth in a safe environment that is conducive to learning.

The program includes intervention techniques based on over 30 years of rigorous research on school discipline within the fields of education, public health, psychology, and criminology. The Best Behavior program components address whole-school, classroom, individual student, and family collaboration practices and are intended to be used in combination with other evidence-based prevention programs, such as the Second Step Violence Prevention Curriculum (Committee for Children, 2002). Representative school team members are trained to develop and implement positive school rules, direct teaching of rules, positive reinforcement systems, data-based decision making at the school level, effective classroom management methods, curriculum adaptation to prevent problem behavior, and functional behavioral assessment and positive behavioral intervention plans. Teams are also coached to integrate Best Behavior with other prevention programs to maximize effectiveness.

What Is the Evidence?

Best Behavior and similar approaches (see Embry & Flannery et al., 1994; Knoff & Batsche, 1995; Taylor-Greene et al., 1997) have been studied by other researchers using similar and identical intervention techniques. The effects of the program are documented in a series of studies implemented by researchers at the University of Oregon (Metzler, Biglan, Rusby, & Sprague, 2001; Sprague, Walker, Golly, et al., 2001; Taylor-Greene et al., 1997, see also *www.pbis.org* for the latest research studies and reports). Studies have shown reductions in office discipline referrals of up to 50% per year, with continued improvement over a 3-year period in schools that sustain the intervention (Irvin et al., 2004). In addition, school staff report greater satisfaction with their work, compared to staff in schools that did not implement Best Behavior. Comparison schools typically show increases or no change in office referrals, along with a general frustration with the school discipline program.

In studies employing the components included in the Best Behavior program, reductions in antisocial behavior (Sprague, Walker, Golly, et al., 2001), vandalism (Mayer, 1995), aggression (Grossman et al., 1997; Lewis, Sugai, & Colvin, 1998), later delinquency (Kellam, Mayer, Rebok, & Hawkins, 1998; O'Donnell et al., 1995), as well as alcohol, tobacco, and other drug use (Biglan, Wang, & Walberg, 2003; O'Donnell et al., 1995) have been documented. Furthermore, positive changes in protective factors such as academic achievement (Kellam et al., 1998; O'Donnell et al., 1995) and school engagement (O'Donnell et al., 1995) have been documented using a schoolwide positive behavior support approach such as Best Behavior in concert with other prevention interventions.

How Is Best Behavior Implemented?

The essential features of the Best Behavior approach should guide implementation of your SWPBS system. We describe the approach here, using illustrative examples. Table 3.1 provides a summary of the "big ideas."

TABLE 3.1. What Does Schoolwide Positive Behavior Support Look Like?

1. Train and support a representative school team (20–30 hours of formal training).
   - Principal actively leads and facilitates the process.
   - Take time to plan, coach, and improve team members' response capabilities.
2. Set and promote schoolwide expectations.
   - Plan to teach expected behavior.
3. Plan to actively supervise students and recognize expected behavior.
4. Define and effectively correct problem behaviors and their consequences for students and staff members.
5. Report data to make decisions and give/seek feedback to/from staff.
   - Office discipline referral patterns (*www.swis.org*)
   - Discipline survey results
   - Changes in academic performance, attendance
   - Student safety surveys
6. Sustain SWPBS practices.
   - Provide ongoing training and coaching
   - Staff meeting discussions
   - Follow-up training

1. *Train and support a representative school team.* Although it would seem ideal to train *all* school staff *all* the time, it is rarely feasible or sustainable to provide training at this level due to cost and logistical concerns. We have found that a group of adults representing all school stakeholders (including students at the secondary level) can learn the key practices of SWPBS and set goals for improvement. The stakeholders can then function as leaders or coaches as they inform their groups of the team activities (e.g., at staff or area meetings) and give support and encouragement during the improvement process. Increasingly, we see district- and statewide initiatives supporting the dissemination of SWPBS training and coaching systems.

While participating in the training and after mastery of the basic material, we recommend that school discipline teams (e.g., building administrator, representative teachers, other stakeholders) meet approximately once per month to review training content, as needed, and to set up a regular process of reviewing and refining the school discipline plan (initial goals are developed during training) and other site-based activities. A format for these meetings should be specified, and each meeting should last between 20 and 60 minutes.

2. *Set and promote schoolwide expectations.* A critical first task for the implementation team is to establish schoolwide teaching of behavioral rules related to student–teacher compliance, peer-to-peer interaction, academic achievement, and academic study skills. We stress the three attributes of *responsible, respectful,* and *safe* behavior and directly teach lessons throughout the year to establish and maintain those patterns of behavior. We also recommend displaying the rules publicly in posters, school newsletters, local media, announcements, assemblies, etc.

3. *Plan to actively supervise students and recognize expected behavior.* Your school will need to establish a consistent system of enforcement, monitoring, and positive reinforcement to enhance the effect of rule teaching and maintain patterns of desired student behavior. Reinforcement systems may include schoolwide token economies in the form of "tickets" stating each school rule and dispersed by all adults in the building. These tokens are to be "backed up" with weekly drawings that bestow rewards for the teachers as well. Each school team should implement the procedures to fit their school improvement plan and specific discipline needs. Figure 3.1 provides a sample token from a school implementing SWPBS practices.

4. *Define and effectively correct problem behaviors and their consequences for students and staff members.* As stated earlier, schools using excessive sanctions experience greater levels of vandalism and other forms of misbehavior (Mayer, 1995; Skiba et al., 1997). Positive reinforcement is more effective than punishment because it does not result in the type of counteraggression or withdrawal (i.e., fight or flight) that punishment can produce and because it does not focus teachers' attention on detecting and correcting rule violations. This is why ignoring minor instances of misbehavior is preferable to attending to it in the hopes of correcting it; we tend to get what we attend to!

Students should observe that the rules are applied fairly. When they feel that rules are unevenly applied, students are more likely to misbehave. Schools with clear rule

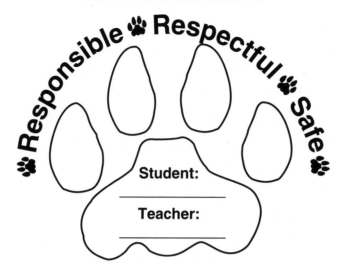

FIGURE 3.1. A sample "good behavior" token.

and reward systems and businesslike corrections and sanctions also experience fewer problems. These schools identify appropriate behavior for students and respond to misbehavior predictably. Students in such schools are clear about expected behavior and learn that there are consequences for misbehavior. When rules are consistent, students develop a respect for them and internalize beliefs that the system of governance works (Bryk & Driscoll, 1988; Gottfredson, 1987; Gottfredson, Gottfredson, & Hybl, 1993).

5. *Report data to make decisions and give/seek feedback to/from staff.* To increase the efficiency of problem solving and to provide recognition for success, we also suggest giving data-based feedback to schools regarding their responses to the: *Best Behavior* survey (Form 3.1) and discipline referral patterns using systems such as the School-Wide Information System (SWIS; developed at the University of Oregon; Sprague, Sugai, Horner, & Walker, 1999; Sugai, Sprague, Horner, & Walker, 2000; *www.swis.org*). Simple bar graphs of each school's performance can be produced and the entire school staff asked to review the data at monthly staff meetings. Staff members can be encouraged to comment on the data and participate in problem-solving discussions to develop action plans during regular school meetings. SWIS is a web-based information system designed to help school personnel use office referral data to design schoolwide and individual student interventions. The three primary components of SWIS are (a) an efficient system for gathering information, (b) a web-based computer application for data entry and report generation, and (c) a practical process for using information for decision-making purposes.

These three components give school personnel the capability to evaluate individual student behavior, the behavior of groups of students, behaviors occurring in specific settings, and behaviors occurring during specific time periods of the school day.

SWIS reports indicate times and locations that are prone to prompt problem behaviors, and allow teachers and administrators to shape schoolwide environments to maximize students' academic and social achievements. Schools are asked to summarize and report the data to school faculty at least monthly. School team members should represent each major stakeholder group. Once implementation goals are set, all stakeholders should receive training and information.

6. *Sustain SWPBS practices*. Research has shown that for intervention to be effective, training and coaching support must be available across the school year. When training or coaching peers, be sure to include rationales, modeling, practice, and coaching. Focus on the data (e.g., office discipline referral patterns) and change your approaches as problems become evident.

As your positive behavior support program progresses, team members can take on the role of trainers and provide technical assistance or help on new methods, coteach expected behavior lessons, and observe or coach colleagues. Some additional types of support to consider include gaining release time for observing or coaching, staff meeting time for discussion and planning, and provision of follow-up training. Finally, additional support needs for your school may include evaluation, "expert" training and consultation, and family liaison.

CONCLUSION

We have described a system for implementing positive behavior support methods at the schoolwide level. It is critical to not view SWPBS as a set of "tricks" but rather as an integrated, sustainable system of supports for students, yourself, and your colleagues.

Research and demonstration efforts are focusing on the long-term impact of SWPBS, and new and improved strategies for implementing universal, selected, and indicated behavior support are emerging. The most important message, however, is that a continuum of behavior support that comprises three very different levels of intervention is needed. The intensity of the intervention must match the intensity of the problem behavior and the complexity of the context in which the problem behavior occurs. SWPBS is the foundation for implementing interventions on all three levels.

Chapter 6 discusses critical issues, procedures, and recommended approaches for meeting the needs of at-risk and severely antisocial students for whom a schoolwide intervention is not sufficient. In addition, a successful demonstration of an alternative school program for this population is described and illustrated. The coordination of schoolwide interventions with specialized accommodations of this type is the key to creating a safe, effective, and inclusive school.

FORM 3.1. *BEST BEHAVIOR* POSITIVE BEHAVIOR SUPPORTS ASSESSMENT

School Name: _____

Date: _____

Your Role (please choose one):

- ❑ Administrator
- ❑ Teacher
- ❑ Classified
- ❑ Special Education Teacher

- ❑ Related Service Provider
- ❑ Parent
- ❑ Student
- ❑ Other _____

School Capacity	In place	Working on it	Not in place	Target as a goal?
1. A representative building leadership team is formed to guide program implementation and evaluation of effectiveness.				
2. The school administrator is an active member of the schoolwide behavior support team.				
3. School personnel (80% or more) have committed to improving school discipline and safety by implementing, supporting, and agreeing to use positive behavior support systems.				
4. A needs assessment has been conducted to guide intervention selection.				
5. An action plan with clear goals and objectives has been developed to improve school discipline.				
6. Regular schoolwide behavior support team meetings are scheduled for training and planning.				
7. Schoolwide behavior support has a budget for rewarding students (and staff), regular team meetings, teaching activities and materials, and data collection and analysis.				

(continued)

School Capacity	In place	Working on it	Not in place	Target as a goal?
Whole-School Behavior Teaching				
8. Three to five schoolwide behavior expectations have been defined (e.g., be safe, respectful, responsible).				
9. Positive behavior expectations have been defined for each school setting (e.g., what does "safe," "respectful," and "responsible" look like in the cafeteria, gym, restrooms).				
10. Lesson plans have been developed for teaching all behavioral expectations in all school settings.				
11. Rules are posted or visible in all school settings (e.g., hallways, classrooms, cafeteria, gym).				
12. Staff have been trained to teach behavioral expectations.				
13. Staff teaches behavioral expectations.				
14. Behavioral expectations for each rule are taught and reviewed at least 10 times per year.				
15. Expected behaviors for each specific setting are taught in that setting at least one time a year.				
Dealing with Problem Behavior				
16. Problem behaviors are clearly defined and explained to all students.				
17. Consequences for problem behaviors are clearly defined and explained to all students.				
18. Staff apply consistent consequences for inappropriate behavior.				
19. Staff consistently correct and reteach students with problem behavior.				
Data-Based Decision Making				
20. Data are collected (e.g., discipline referrals, surveys) to guide decision making.				

(continued)

71

School Capacity	In place	Working on it	Not in place	Target as a goal?
21. Data are regularly summarized (e.g., at least monthly) by discipline/behavior support team.				
22. Staff receive regular (e.g., at least monthly) reports on key discipline outcomes (e.g., information about referrals, suspensions).				
23. Intervention decisions and strategies are evaluated regularly (e.g., at least once per term) based on behavior data.				
Classroom Management				
24. The school has defined systems of classroom behavior management.				
25. Curriculum and instruction match student ability; students have high rates of academic success (75%+ correct).				
26. Transitions within classrooms, between activities, and between settings are planned for, taught to students, well-established, and orderly.				
Individual Student Support				
27. Teachers can easily get assistance with problem students in their classroom.				
28. Behavioral assessments are used to identify students with problem behavior.				
29. A behavior support team attends promptly (within 2 school days) when a student exhibits chronic problem behavior.				
30. Teachers are trained in, and use, effective methods to prevent behavioral escalation.				
31. Teachers are trained in functional behavioral assessment and positive behavioral intervention for students with chronic problem behavior.				

(continued)

School Capacity	In place	Working on it	Not in place	Target as a goal?
Family Support and Collaboration				
32. Families are active participants in supporting whole-school discipline systems.				
33. The school reinforces good parenting practices by providing information and support to families.				
34. The school has defined systems for maintaining regular, positive contacts with families.				
35. At least one parent is a member of the whole-school positive discipline team.				
36. There are adequate staff present on playgrounds, during recess and free time, and in other common areas to effectively supervise the number of students present.				
37. A system of positive reinforcement is in place in all common area settings.				
38. Recess, free time, playground, and/or common areas are easily observable (i.e., unobstructed views) from any given position in the area.				
39. Supervisors maintain close contact with students in all recess, free time, playground, and/or common areas.				
40. Playground, recess, and recreational equipment are safe.				
41. Access to and from the playground, recess, and free-time areas is supervised.				
42. Formal emergency or crisis procedures for students and staff on playgrounds and in recess and other common areas have been developed and are practiced at least twice a year.				
43. Common area supervision staff have been trained in active supervision techniques and methods this year.				

(continued)

FORM 3.1. *(page 5 of 6)*

School Capacity	In place	Working on it	Not in place	Target as a goal?
44. A system for addressing minor problem behavior in recess, playground, and common areas is in place and practiced by common area supervision staff.				
45. A system for addressing serious or major problem behavior in recess, playground, and common areas is in place and practiced by all common area supervision staff.				
46. Off-limits areas are clearly identified, taught to students and staff, and known by all.				
47. All staff have received training in active supervision of common areas.				

(continued)

FORM 3.1. *(page 6 of 6)*

Goals

Review the results of your self-assessment and identify the top three or four priorities for improvement of school discipline systems. List a clear goal statement and then use the box on the right to set concrete action steps.

Improvement Goal	Action Steps
Goal 1:	
Goal 2:	
Goal 3:	
Goal 4:	

4

Bullying and Peer-Based Harassment in Schools

Current Status, Influencing Factors, and Identification Methods

with STEPHEN G. SMITH

No matter what their experiences or background in growing up, most adults can remember at least one or two occasions during childhood where they were picked on, made fun of in front of peers, humiliated in some way, threatened, intimidated, or perhaps even beaten up. Most can clearly recall the student or students who did these things as well as details and circumstances surrounding the incident, even though they may not be able to remember much else from this period in their lives. Not surprisingly, such unpleasant situations are often initiated and sustained by the student or students who are commonly known as school bullies.

Nearly everyone who has attended school has had some experience with the schoolyard bully. In the vast majority of cases, such experience tends to be negative and emotionally searing, whether it plays out directly or indirectly. Perhaps that student picked on them or others, called them names, teased them, or somehow embarrassed them in public. Maybe the bully took something from them or deliberately broke a prized possession just to be mean—or simply because the bully knew he or she could do it. Overt, painful, and intimidating events of this nature are more likely characteristic of boys than girls (Espelage & Swearer, 2003), and they tend to occur in school settings where there is limited adult supervision and monitoring to prevent

76

them. Nevertheless, girls also engage in bullying and peer harassment of each other at rates that some researchers say approximately equal those of boys (Crick & Grotpeter, 1995). However, their bullying is typically expressed in more subtle behavioral forms known as relational (or social) aggression; it is much more covert in nature and can occur in any setting at basically any time. Those engaged in relational aggression tend to exclude others from activities, damage reputations through backbiting, tell lies, and spread rumors, try to ruin existing friendships through alienation, and engage in social manipulation and discrimination of others for indefensible reasons. Typically girls do not display the kind of overt "in-your-face" bullying that is identified as characteristic of boys. It should be stressed, however, that both genders engage in overt (direct, physical) and covert (indirect, social) bullying and harassment behavior. In the past it seemed that male bullying consisted mostly of overt behaviors and female bullying was largely confined to covert behaviors. Today, this division along gender lines seems to be blurring in society, and especially in schools. It is obvious from media accounts, school reports, and legal actions that female aggression and violence are occurring on a daily basis. Likewise, any boy in school will tell you that boys regularly engage in social bullying. The upshot is that both types of bullying and harassment can be extremely damaging to the victim and the perpetrators (i.e., long-term social and academic outcomes for bullies are very negative; Graham & Juvonen, 2001).

Students grow up and leave school—including those mean kids of long ago, but in a certain sense the bully never actually grows up; he or she still bullies, harasses, and intimidates others. Little has changed over the years in this regard, with the possible exception that things may have gotten measurably worse—especially within the context of schooling. Certainly, there is now broad concern over this issue by educators in response to such factors as court decisions, the complaints and actions of parents of victimized children, and the distinct possibility that bullying and peer harassment have become more invasive, widespread, and more public. In a CNN interview, the U.S. Surgeon General recently declared that bullying and peer harassment are public health problems that require federal attention and intervention in order for them to be solved. The federal government is in the process of initiating a national, anti-bullying campaign to raise public awareness and to lay the foundation for a broad-based response to this type of youth victimization.

THE CURRENT LANDSCAPE OF SCHOOL-BASED BULLYING AND PEER HARASSMENT

Espelage and Swearer (2003) have recently noted that bullying and harassment by peers are now common occurrences in most U.S. schools. These toxic social events are recognized as problems worldwide requiring adult attention and intervention. Numerous scholars and experts on bullying have described the international attention that has been focused on these problems and have also noted the efforts of countries outside the United States to document bullying and harassment problems. Societies as culturally different from each other as South Africa, Japan, Norway, Britain, and Canada all report concerns about bullying and harassment among their youth.

Limber and Small (2003) cite empirical evidence showing that bullying and harassment pose very serious psychological and behavioral risks for victims and bullies alike, and they argue that these events can have a serious, negative impact on the climate and social ecology of schools. All of our collective experience with antisocial behavior patterns, school violence, and peer relations validates these observations. Aside from the tragedy of school shootings, severe bullying, in our view, is one of *the* most violent acts that occurs on school grounds.

This chapter reviews the general characteristics, dynamics, and prevalence of the bully/victim problem in today's schools. We discuss legal and policy implications as well as methods for screening and identifying bullies and their victims. Chapter 5 describes recommended solutions and prevention strategies.

THE CHARACTERISTICS AND CRITICAL FEATURES OF BULLYING AND HARASSMENT IN TODAY'S SCHOOLS

The Relationship of Bullying and Harassment to Antisocial Behavior

There are varied, overlapping, and sometimes conflicting characterizations of bullying and harassment in the professional literature. Although bullying and harassment have social, political, and legal implications, the specific forms of negative and aggressive behavior involved in bullying and harassment are broadly recognized as examples of *antisocial behavior,* a term that refers to the consistent violation of social norms by at-risk individuals across a range of settings (Simcha-Fagan, Langner, Gersten, & Eisenberg, 1975; Smith & Sprague, 2003). This is not to say, however, that the students who engage in bullying and harassment in school are necessarily diagnosed as antisocial bullies and harassers. They are considered aggressive, but they are not invariably labeled as violent or antisocial because their bullying and harassing activities are frequently circumscribed, contained within narrow contexts and windows of time, and are most often not physically threatening. In addition, students who frequently bully and harass others may not display the characteristics of antisocial behavior, as it has been described in the literature (Reid, Patterson, & Snyder, 2002; Walker, Ramsey, & Gresham, 2004). A key difference between behavior that is defined as antisocial and that which is considered bullying and harassment is the persistent and recurring nature of the behavioral cycle that repeatedly occurs between perpetrators and their familiar, targeted victims. In contrast, youth identified as classically antisocial tend to direct their aggression and antisocial behavior in a largely random fashion and toward large pools of potential targets (victims) among peers and adults. Behaviors identified as belonging to bullying and harassment are much more likely to be directed toward specific individuals, to occur within contexts where they have been in evidence previously and where they are very common occurrences, and in settings that are not easily or regularly accessible to adult monitoring.

It is well documented that certain individuals within the peer group may have much higher probabilities of being bullied and harassed than others due to their attributes (e.g., physical appearance, size, unusual name) and/or behavioral characteristics (e.g., atypical behavior, displaying either submissive or provocative responses in relation to acts of bullying/harassment; see Graham & Juvonen, 2001). Typically, bullies tend to repeatedly seek out certain individuals as victims because (1) the behavioral and psychological risks associated with humiliating and torturing these target students are quite low; (2) target victims, as noted, tend to reinforce the bully's behavior through their responses to it; and (3) peers who bully and harass others often gain social status and behavioral influence with their peers through these acts. In addition, some bullies enjoy high social status and are popular with peers; this small subset of popular students choose to use their social status as a license to taunt and psychologically torture certain peers (Rodkin & Hodges, 2003). Intervening successfully with bullying and harassing students poses a daunting challenge for educators and requires attention to both victimizers and their victims as well as the supportive roles played by nonparticipating members of the peer group (e.g., bystanders, peers who distance themselves from bullying, defenders of the victim; see Snell, MacKenzie, & Frey, 2002).

Interpersonal Violence as a Correlate of Severe Bullying

Nansel, Overpeck, Haynie, Ruan, and Scheidt (2003) recently reported a study of the relationship between severe forms of bullying within and outside school settings and violence among U.S. youth. These authors examined this relationship for both bullies and their victims in a cross-sectional sample of 15,686 participating students. The sample consisted of students in the grade 6–10 range and included students attending public, private, and parochial schools. The study was part of a World Health Organization (WHO) investigation of health risk behavior involving adolescents from 30 participating countries. Students in the sample responded to the WHO Health Behavior in School-Aged Children Survey that included questions on such violence indicators as weapons carrying, frequent fighting, and reports of injuries received from fighting. Results of this study showed consistent relationships between bullying and interpersonal violence. Involvement in violence-related behavior ranged from 13 to 23% of boys and from 4 to 11% of girls. Both bullying others and being bullied were related to higher frequencies of violence, with greater odds of involvement occurring for bullying others than being bullied. In addition, there were greater odds of involvement in violence for bullying that took place away from school than within school. The odds ratio for weapons carrying associated with being bullied weekly in school was 1.5; for bullying others in school, 2.6; for being bullied away from school, 4.1; and for bullying others away from school, 5.9. It is likely that some of the bullying victims in this study were carrying weapons for their own protection, with still others carrying weapons who were both bullies and victims of bullying. These results highlight the socially toxic conditions associated with bullying and harassment of peers and help document the importance of schools and parents forging partnerships that will effectively address them early on in children's development.

State Legislation and Definitions of Bullying

There is a growing awareness in the United States and other countries that preventing and addressing bullying and harassment in schools has become a school responsibility under the law—and rightly so, in our view. Limber and Small (2003), in a comprehensive review of federal and state legislation on bullying, note that state laws are much more likely than federal initiatives to directly influence school district policies and practices on bullying. However, federal court decisions have been instrumental in supplying the necessary mandates for states and schools to begin reducing and eliminating their problems with bullying and harassment.

A recent Supreme Court decision found in favor of a female student (*Davis v. Monroe County Board of Education*, 1999) who had sued her school district for its failure to take action in response to the unrelenting bullying, sexual harassment, and emotional victimization that she had consistently experienced at the hands of peers. This decision has had a far-reaching impact and has served notice to schools that they must actively address the issue of school bullying and harassment or face the very real possibility of serious legal consequences. Other seminal events in this context, such as the Casey Woodruff case (Seale, 2002), in which elementary-age students were caught on school district video in the act of brutalizing a fellow student on a bus while the driver was present and the bus was stopped, serve to illustrate the severity and pervasiveness of this problem in our schools. Our society is becoming highly sensitized to this issue and its ramifications through such media exposure.

Three primary domains for defining bullying have relevance for the school environment and the way in which this problem is addressed by school personnel:

1. Federal, state, and local law and statute
2. State-level departments of education and school district policies
3. Clinical practice and research

Governmental and Educational Definitions

The first two definitional approaches noted above are important because they provide both a legal and policy basis for defining unacceptable behavior within the school setting. Conversely, clinical and research-based definitions of bullying and harassment provide a conceptual and empirical basis for the development of law, statute, and policy as well as a basis for the development and implementation of effective intervention programs.

A number of states have established legislation and policies regarding bullying that are designed to address this behavior within public school settings. Fifteen states have enacted such legislation; others are in the process and will soon pass such legislation; and still others are strongly considering its development and passage. These laws, statutes, and policies are important to educators because (1) they define the specific behavior(s) of concern in legal terms, (2) they outline and delineate the legal requirements for compliance with the statute, law, or policy, and (3) they may also provide guidelines on how to achieve compliance and thereby indemnify responsible parties (in this case, schools and school personnel).

Laws and policies addressing bullying, harassment, and intimidation are "a work in progress" and are highly variable across states and local agencies. A review of several states' laws, statutes, and policies concerning bullying and harassment in school reveals common features: 9 of the 15 states examined currently have legislation defining bullying in their laws; the remainder have deferred this task to state Departments of Education and local school districts (see Limber & Small, 2003).

Clinical and Research Definitions

Walker, Ramsey, and Gresham (2004) define bullying as a form of peer-related antisocial behavior that "involves coercion, intimidation, and threats to one's safety or well being" (p. 238). Similarly, Olweus (1996) defines bullying as the recurring exposure, over time, to negative actions by one or more others. Snell et al. (2002) identify three critical features that most definitions of bullying have in common: (1) there is a perceived power imbalance between perpetrator and victim involving factors such as physical size, age, peer or social support, and social status; (2) there is intent to harm or injure; and (3) it is a repeated, often chronic, antisocial activity involving a specific targeted person.

Many bullying definitions include components that are difficult to observe and document, such as "intent," "social capital," "social status," and "power imbalance." One of the reasons bullying and harassment are so difficult to cope with in schools is that their covert nature and the often subtle forms of behavior through which they are expressed make them very difficult to monitor and detect. It is incumbent upon those who are responsible for the security and welfare of students that they institute effective methods for determining if and when a bullying or harassment situation exists; and if so, to make the necessary investments and implement measures and methods that will effectively address it.

For educators, a useful working definition of bullying and harassment is suggested as follows: Bullying and harassing interactions involve the *apparent* (i.e., as might be determined by any reasonable person) intent to physically, socially, or mentally harm the target victim(s) and may include (1) physical and/or verbal threats or assaults, (2) offensive and/or threatening gestures and facial expressions, (3) verbal, physical, or social intimidation, and (4) social exclusion from groups and friends. Furthermore, bullying and harassment (5) nearly always involve an apparent power imbalance between the bully/harasser and the victim(s), (6) occur repeatedly over time, and (7) often involve the same students. This gender-neutral definition clearly specifies the forms of peer-to-peer interactive behavior that are unacceptable in school. It is essential that students, staff, administrators and parents all become aware of this definition as a key first step in raising awareness about the unacceptability of this form of behavior.

Types of Bullying

There are three main types of bullying, as described by Olweus (1993, 1994): *direct bullying*, consisting of overt, relatively open attacks on the intended victim; *indirect bullying*, consisting of covert actions intended to socially isolate or exclude the victim from groups and friends; and *passive bullying*, which refers to the followers (henchmen) who lend peer support for a leader involved in bullying or harassment. As noted earlier, direct bullying is most often associated with boys, whereas indirect bullying is most often associated with girls—although not exclusively (Olweus, 1996). Direct bullying is a public event, involves overt actions designed to intimidate or humiliate the victim, and the impact of the bullying is immediate and powerful. Typically, the victim knows the victimizer in cases of direct bullying. In contrast, the taunting actions involved in indirect bullying are often covert and the target victim may not even be aware that they are happening—as in the case of relational aggression wherein an individual's reputation is "trashed" (See Crick & Grotpeter, 1995). The perpetrator is often hidden or unknown to the victim, has hostile intentions, and the involved actions typically have a delayed but harmful impact on the victim.

Prevalence of Bullying in Schools

Olweus (1994, 1996) reported on European studies of the prevalence of school-based bullying conducted in concert with the development and implementation of his anti-bullying intervention (the Bullying Prevention Program; see the Blueprint Series Publication of the Center for the Study and Prevention of Violence, University of Colorado at Boulder; Mihalic, Irwin, Elliott, Fagan, & Hansen, 2001). He found that 7–9% of children surveyed in grades 1–9 had bullied other students with some regularity, and about 5% of surveyed students were involved in serious bullying at least once a week. Students as victims accounted for 9% of all students surveyed, and 17% of these victims reported acting as *both* bully and victim. Students in the lower grades (1st, 2nd, 3rd, and 4th) reported experiencing victimization at a greater rate than students in the higher grades (7th, 8th, and 9th). Olweus estimates that the actual figures may be somewhat higher, as underreporting of bullying is a common occurrence in European schools due to the negative social stigma attached to its reporting by students. Other early studies (Hoover, Oliver, & Hazler, 1992) found that up to 75% of the students surveyed reported being victimized and as many as 14% of all students surveyed had suffered severe trauma as a result.

In the United States, studies of the prevalence of bullying in schools report rates that vary widely, and many of the frequencies exceed those reported by Olweus for European schools. It is estimated that approximately 160,000 U.S. students miss school each day due to bullying and harassment. Bullying in our schools appears to be quite common, with 1 in 4 students in grades 4–6 reporting that they are bullied regularly, and 1 in 10 who say they are bullied weekly. It appears that approximately 6–10% of U.S. students are chronically bullied and have a much higher likelihood of being selected as victims than their peers. More of these chronic victims are reported at the elementary level than at middle or high school. Approximately 6% of school-age students are bully victims *and* victimizers of others (Walker, Ramsey, & Gresham, 2004).

Hoover et al. (1992) reported a study of bullying among junior high and high school students in a series of Midwestern towns and found that 88% of students had observed instances of bullying and 77% of students reported being a victim of bullying at some point during their school careers. Nansel et al. (2001) found that a total of 29.9% of their 15,000-plus student sample indicated frequent involvement in bullying episodes; 13% reported acting as a bully, 10.6% said they were victims, and 6% indicated they had been both bully and victim. Kochenderfer and Ladd (1996, 1997) interviewed 200 boys and girls in kindergarten and found that 18% reported being victims of bullying at this early age!

Recent surveys (Smith & Sprague, 2001; 2003; Smith, Sprague, Myers, & Anderson, 2000) of elementary, middle, and high school students in Oregon seem to support the presence of higher rates of bullying and harassment. In school-administered student surveys of elementary students in third, fourth, and fifth grade, these authors found that 93% had witnessed a peer or group of peers being mean to another student, and 81% had been present when a peer or group of peers had physically assaulted another student while at school. These statistics for the state of Oregon assume greater meaning when viewed in light of findings from the 1999 Youth Risk Behavior Survey (YRBS; see the YRBS website: *www.cdc.gov/ HealthyYouth/yrbs/index.htm*). In this national survey of 9th-, 10th-, 11th-, and 12th-grade students, 14.2% of respondents reported having been in a physical fight on school property in the past year, and 7.7% reported that they had been threatened or injured with a weapon on school property two or more times during the preceding 12 months. In addition, 5.2% of respondents reported having missed two or more days of school during the preceding 30 days because they had felt unsafe at school or when traveling to or from school. In the U.S. Secret Service analysis of the characteristics of school shooters, it was found that the most common shared characteristic of these youth was having been the target of a school bully; 71% of them reported being so victimized (Fein et al., 2002).

Nansel et al. (2003) forcefully make the case that bullying and harassment should not be considered normative in *any* setting, regardless of their frequency of occurrence. In our view, they are destructive processes and are *not* a rite of passage that all children should be expected to endure as part of "growing up." Bullies are victimizers of others and also victims of their own behavior. The long-term consequences of chronically engaging in bullying behavior can be quite destructive socially and in terms of quality of life. The next section describes correlates and outcomes associated with bullies and their victims.

THE SOCIAL DYNAMICS OF BULLYING AND PEER HARASSMENT

Olweus (2001) has developed one of the most comprehensive and widely referenced conceptualizations of bullying. Figure 4.1 displays this conceptual model in terms of the various roles and reactions that youth characteristically assume in acute bullying situations. It is most important that the students who assume and display these roles and reactions be identified as part of developing any effective solution to the problems of peer harassment. These roles and reactions have everything to do with the control and prevention of peer harassment processes.

Based on his research in Norwegian schools, Olweus (1993, 1996) reported that

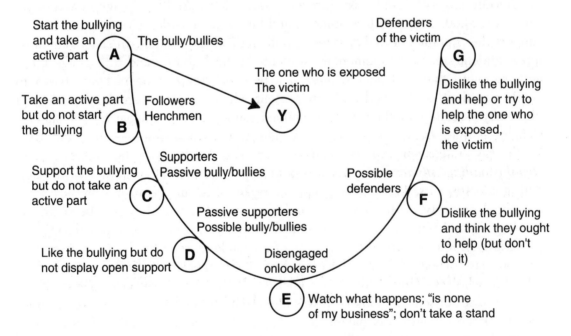

FIGURE 4.1. The bullying circle: Students' modes of reaction/roles in an acute bullying situation. From Olweus, Limber, and Mihalic (2000). Copyright 2000 by the Institute of Behavioral Science, Regents of the University of Colorado. Reprinted by permission.

bullies are likely to be physically stronger than their typical peer, average to just below average in popularity, accompanied by one or two henchmen (i.e., passive bullies), and generally older than their victims. In contrast, victims are likely to be younger, physically weaker, cautious, shy and quiet, and less popular than either bullies or normal students. Walker, Ramsey, and Gresham (2004) describe bullies as having primarily *externalizing* (defined as an excess of behavior) behavioral profiles characterized by a much higher-than-normal rate of negative social behavior toward their peers. These students are often labeled as aggressive toward others and they tend to affiliate with peers who share their attitudes, beliefs, and actions. Those students who are likely to be targeted as victims are commonly described as having primarily *internalizing* (defined as a deficit in behavior and skill level) behavioral profiles characterized by a very low level of negative social behavior with their peers. They also spend large amounts of time alone compared to normal, socially adaptable students. Olweus (1996) has identified a second type of victim as "provocative"; this is the student who gets angry and upset and tends to fight back or try to extract revenge in response to bullying or taunts by peers. Both types of victims are harassed and victimized at much higher-than-normal rates by peers (see Juvonen & Graham, 2001).

Students who establish a pattern of passive/submissive responding to bullying and harassment may be victimized frequently and by a significant number of their peers, as opportunities allow. These unfortunate students often lack the social skills and peer status necessary to fend off attacks by fellow students and to prevent their appearance as a relatively risk-free target for bullying and harassment. Target victims who are ineffective in their aggressive behavior and who display provocative responses to peer taunts are often seen as inviting peer bullying and harassment (Perry, Hodges, & Egan, 2001). Provocative students may be targeted for victimization by engaging in obnoxious, irritating, or other annoying behaviors in common social situations, marking them as "a good tease." A subset of students becomes involved in a recurring bully/victim cycle, wherein these students assume both bully and victim roles. An even smaller subset of frequently victimized students appears to expect to be bullied by peers and are known to actually prompt peer bullies to taunt them on occasion (Juvonen & Graham, 2001; Olweus, 1991, 1993, 1996; Walker, Severson, & Feil, 1995; Patterson, Reid, & Dishion, 1992; Colvin, Sugai, Good, & Lee, 1997; Smith & Sprague, 2003; Snell et al., 2002).

COMMON ATTRIBUTES AND BEHAVIORAL CHARACTERISTICS OF BULLIES AND THEIR VICTIMS: WHAT DO THEY LOOK LIKE?

As noted, overt bullying has been mainly associated with males and covert bullying has been mostly associated with females (Crick & Grotpeter, 1995; Olweus, 1996). Neither gender nor age, however, is a valid predictor of the onset and expression of bullying and harassment. In today's schools, increasing numbers of female students engage in direct and overt forms of bullying and harassment, just as indirect, covert bullying and harassment are practiced with greater frequency by male students. However, in general, it can be said that male bullies have a more positive attitude toward violence, are more impulsive, typically display a strong need to dominate others, seem to have little empathy for others, and often display aggressive reaction patterns to difficult social situations. They characteristically use a perceived advantage in physical strength, weapons, and/or peer supports to menace, intimidate, and abuse their victims (Nansel et al., 2003; Olweus, 1996). Female bullies tend to use covert, nonphysical, nonconfrontational methods of harassment to abuse their victims. These bullies routinely display a strong need to socially dominate others, to be the center of attention of a core group of peers, to exclude others from their core group, to exhibit aggressive and socially reactive behavior patterns, and they display little empathy or caring toward others in certain situations (Olweus, 1996). Female bullies frequently spread destructive, damaging rumors or lies about targets among their peers; this practice becomes more damaging and frequent as females make the transition into adolescence (Juvonen & Graham, 2001).

High levels of anger seem to be a strong precursor and predictor of bullying in both sexes (Bosworth, Espelage, & Simon, 1999; Espelage, Bosworth, & Simon, 2001) leading Espelage and Swearer (2003) to speculate that anger-management training may be an important intervention component in addressing bullying. Depressive symptoms are commonly seen in both male and female victims. Clinical levels of depression have also been found in both male and female victimizers of others (Callaghan & Joseph, 1995). A mixture of anger, aggression, and depression is a dangerous combination and can lead to highly destructive outcomes for victims and bullies alike.

Victims, both male and female, tend to have characteristics that set them apart from the average or normal student. *Passive/submissive* victims act more insecure, anxious, cautious, and sensitive than do students in general (Olweus, 1996). They are more withdrawing and more easily intimidated than normal students (Juvonen & Graham, 2001). When attacked by peers, they tend to react by crying, submitting and withdrawing. These chronic and perpetual victims are prone to low self-esteem, as reflected in their high rates of social and academic failure, and in their self-reports they note that they feel stupid, ashamed, incompetent, and unattractive. This type of victim is characterized by "a submissive reaction pattern combined (in the case of boys) with physical weakness" (Olweus, 1996, p. 18).

Provocative victims, on the other hand, are characterized by a combination of both aggressive and anxious reaction patterns, and they seek to retaliate toward peers who taunt them—usually ineffectually (Olweus, 1996; Perry, Perry, & Kennedy, 1992). These students are often tense, irritating to those around them, emotionally labile, overly active and restless, ineffective in self-regulation, and have problems with concentration (Olweus, 1996). Aggressive victims are also highly disliked by their peers and frequently appear in the socially rejected category of peer sociometric assessments (Kupersmidt, Patterson, & Eickholt (1989). This dislike doubtless contributes to peers' judgments that many provocative victims deserve the bullying and harassment treatment they receive (Schwartz, Proctor, & Chen, 2001). As a result, few peers are willing to defend them and come to their aid during instances of bullying and harassment (Graham & Juvonen, 2001).

The problem dynamics presented by bully/submissive victim interactions can differ greatly from the problem dynamics presented by bully/provocative victim interactions. The *bully/submissive victim* context may be exacerbated both by the perpetrator's perception of the ease and risk-free features of the social situation, based on previous experience, along with the victims' historical inability or unwillingness to resist the bullying and to defend themselves. The submissive victim typically presents few, if any, effective social skills that might enable either active or passive resistance to bullying and harassment by others. When confronted with bullying and harassment challenges, the submissive victim may even perceive the interaction to be part of a normal social relationship.

In *bully/provocative victim* situations, the victim typically exhibits a range of irritating, obnoxious, and atypical personal and social attributes, including poor personal hygiene, unusual clothing, deviant humor, poor interpersonal skills, generally underdeveloped coping skills, use of aggressive tactics that are usually ineffective in achieving intended outcomes, and difficulty in developing and sustaining peer relationships and friendships. The student likely to be characterized as a provocative victim may also be one whom even adults have difficulty liking and accepting. Some of these children are outgoing, assertive, academically skilled, and come from stable home environments; others are what educators typically identify as "needy," bothersome, overly dependent, and/or socially maladjusted. Their difficulties may stem from a range of environmental vulnerabilities, such as poverty, a dysfunctional home life, and social, emotional, and mental health problems that impede their ability to develop and maintain satisfactory, productive, and lasting interpersonal relationships. There is even evidence that family dynamics and unhealthy parenting practices can influence a child's likelihood of being a victim of bullying and harassment at school (see Perry et al., 2001). As noted earlier, both submissive and provocative victims tend to exhibit divergent behavioral reactions that characteristically invite bullying and harassment from peers and ultimately lead to a greater likelihood of their future occurrence.

VIEWS OF BULLYING AND HARASSMENT BY VICTIMS AND THEIR PEERS

When interviewed, many victims of bullying and harassment tend to blame themselves and assume responsibility for the occurrence of these events. Janoff-Bulman (1979) has distinguished between behavioral and characterological self-blame—a differentiation that has substantial relevance to understanding how victims rationalize their frequent victimization at the hands of their peers. When behavioral self-blame is the victim's pattern, the victim assumes he or she did something (or failed to do something) that caused the bullying/harassment to occur; thus, these events happened for identifiable reasons and were to be expected, in a sense. In contrast, with characterological self-blame, the bullying and harassment are assumed by victims to occur because of some attribute or attributes intrinsic to them (i.e., "It must be something about me that causes it"). With behavioral self-blame, the victim has implicit control over whether or not victimization occurs (by reframing the behavior believed to incite it), whereas with characterological self-blame, the victimization is regarded as being beyond the person's control or influence ("It's just how I *am*"). Graham and Juvonen (2001) document empirical evidence that shows that individuals who make characterological self-attributions are more depressed, have lower self-esteem, and are more poorly adjusted than those who attribute the victimization to behavioral factors (Frazier, 1990; Janoff-Bulman (1979). A consistent finding in the research on peer-based victimization is that victims tend to be socially rejected by their peers, regardless of whether they are viewed as provocative or submissive. As a rule, peers tend to show little empathy or concern for victims of bullying and harassment; many adolescents, in fact, view them as deserving of their fate and are reluctant to come to their rescue (Salmivalli, 2001). In other instances, observers and bystanders do nothing and rationalize it by attributing the bullying and harassment to inherent characteristics of the aggressor (see Graham & Juvonen, 2001).

These findings have important implications for the prevention and remediation of bullying/harassment problems in schools. Members of the peer group have to play key participating and supportive roles in school-based interventions for bully-proofing efforts to be successful. The attitudes and behavioral inclinations of peers toward victims, as noted above, should be addressed as part of any comprehensive intervention to make school a bully-free zone.

PERSONAL QUALITIES AS DETERMINANTS OF VICTIMIZATION BY PEERS

Perry et al. (2001) have recently reviewed the evidence regarding patterns of chronic victimization of peers. Such victimization can begin as early as preschool age and extend throughout the K–12 age–grade range. These authors note that personal, peer relational, and family relational factors all influence the likelihood of children being victimized by peers and that risk and protective factors operate within each domain. For example, children who show known vulnerabilities (risk factors) to bullying, such as physical weakness, are less likely to be victimized if they are fortunate enough to have formed solid friendships and support systems (a protective factor) within the peer group.

In the personal realm, research by Olweus has shown that certain individuals maintain relatively stable attributes and characteristics that cause them to attract bullying and harassment from peers (Olweus, 1978; Perry et al., 2001). For example, some students who change classrooms and even schools continue to experience chronic harassment at the hands of their peers, indicating that they carry with them personal qualities and perhaps expectations that lead to bullying and harassment. Perry et al. (2001) have identified personal qualities, including physical attributes, behavioral attributes, and social–cognitive factors, that contribute to the likelihood of being victimized by peers.

Physical attributes include salient atypical characteristics, such as obesity, wearing glasses, having speech problems, being clumsy, or having an obvious disabling condition. These attributes may be more likely to prompt mean-spirited teasing than bullying; however, they can establish the child as a target of frequent peer harassment. Obvious physical weakness (especially among boys) is associated with frequent bullying and victimization; it sends a message that the target individual can be intimidated and threatened with impunity as he or she likely is incapable of effective self-defense.

Behavioral attributes that may invite chronic victimization include submissive behavior that tends to end the harassment episode but also serves to encourage the attacker's behavior over the long term. In contrast, children who actively resist the attacker tend to become angry, lose the ability to control their emotions, and engage in extended arguments and confrontations that also increase the likelihood of future attacks. The victim often leaves this situation in tears, while muttering threats about extracting revenge. Both types of resistance illustrate serious deficits in the social skills required to negotiate complex peer group dynamics.

A number of researchers on bullying and harassment have concluded that victims have social information deficits and poor problem-solving capacities that impair their ability to anticipate, prevent, and ward off attacks from peers. Victims (both passive and provocative) also suffer from low self-esteem and poor self-concepts. Egan and Perry (1998) found that physical weakness and poor social skills (risk factors) are less likely to lead to victimization among children who have a strong sense of self (protective factor).

The interaction between the personal qualities of an individual and the social ecology of the myriad situations and settings in which they operate can become extremely complex when bullying and harassment are involved. Many of these dynamics are not open to, or accessible by, adults (parents, teachers) and play out in very destructive ways. Understanding these complex phenomena, in our view, requires adoption of a social–ecological model that examines the individual's characteristics and behavior in relation to the demands, opportunities, resources, and challenges present in specific settings (primarily the school and home environments). A theoretical model of this type should also serve as a foundation for investigation of these phenomena (Bronfen-brenner, 1979; Espelage & Swearer, 2003; Romer & Heller, 1983).

THE INFLUENCE OF SOCIAL CONTEXT
ON BULLYING DYNAMICS

There are three primary settings and correlated social contexts that influence the dynamics involving bullies and their victims: (1) the family situation and associated parenting practices, (2) free play settings (i.e., the playground) and peer relations, and (3) classroom settings and the teacher. Substantial research has been conducted on the impact of each of these influencing factors on the behavior of bullies and victims, and both direct and indirect effects have been documented. Findings from these three settings and contexts are discussed below.

The Family Situation and Associated Parenting Practices

Attachment histories with parents are an important influence on whether a child later becomes a target for victimization by peers in school settings. Perry et al. (2001) cite evidence that preschool and elementary-age children who have histories of insecure attachment during infancy are more likely than children with secure attachment histories to be targets of peer aggression (Jacobson & Willie, 1986; Troy & Stroufe, 1987). Research shows that victims commonly have attachment problems with the mother (e.g., insecure attachment; Rodkin & Hodges, 2003; Troy & Stroufe, 1987).

Children with anxious/resistant attachment disorders are easily upset by relatively innocuous situations and events, frequently experience separation anxiety, are overly dependent on the parent, and are not easily calmed when upset (Perry et al., 2001). Rodkin and Hodges (2003) describe two types of insecure attachment: avoidant and preoccupied. *Avoidant attachment* is associated with aggression and externalizing behavior problems; *preoccupied attachment* is predictive of victimization and internalizing behavior problems (Hodges, Finnegan, & Perry, 1999). Maternal overprotectiveness and an intensely close maternal relationship predict peer victimization, especially among boys; excessive parental demands, coercion, and threats of rejection are linked to victimization among girls. Child abuse has also been associated with victimization by peers (Shield, Cicchetti, & Ryan, 1994).

Perry et al. (2001) have identified three types of parenting practices that are associated with victimization by peers: (1) intrusive and overprotective parenting that impairs development of the child's autonomy; (2) parental overcontrol that is manipulative and undermines the child's self-confidence; and (3) coercive parenting practices (e.g., rejection, verbal or physical attacks, threats, harsh discipline) that contribute both to aggression *and* victimization in the child. It is possible that this latter form of parenting is associated with the dual bully/victim role some children manifest.

It is remarkable, in one sense, that parenting practices from earliest infancy can have such far-reaching influences on peer relations, years later, to shape a child as a likely victim of peer-based harassment and/or as a victimizer of others. However, the social context provided by the family situation and the behavior of parents clearly constitute perhaps the most powerful influence on how children develop and ultimately "turn out" (Reid, 2002).

Free Play Settings and Peer Relations

The playground is a setting in which peer-group dynamics play out in their purest, most unconstrained fashion of all school environs. As a rule, these settings are inadequately supervised by adults, and playground supervisors have very little influence or control over what takes place in them. The unstructured nature of the playground and its relatively supervision-poor status provide many opportunities for peer victimization. Among younger children, the majority of fights, bullying, and sexual harassment episodes occur on the playground, and most school injuries can also be traced to this setting (Craig & Pepler, 1997; Leff, Power, Costigan, & Manz, 2003). When asked what schools can do to reduce bullying and to make schools safer, students typically respond with advice to have a greater adult presence in low-traffic areas of the school.

Leff et al. (2003) note that there is an ongoing debate about the merits of recess and whether it should even continue to be part of the regular school day. However, on balance, the advantages of recess seem to clearly outweigh its negative features. Recess is one of the few settings that peers can claim as their own; it affords important opportunities for developing peer-related social skills; and it provides a setting for recruiting friendships and social support networks (Pellegrini, 2001).

Affiliation with antisocial groups ranks as a key accelerator of violent responses among at-risk youth (American Psychological Association, 1993). Patterson and his colleagues have documented the role of deviant peer-group affiliation along the path to delinquency: Sociometric assessments indicate that antisocial children tend to pick other antisocial children in school as their best friends (Patterson et al., 1992). Such group bonding and social cohesion provide a powerful context for socialization toward deviance, including bullying and harassment of peers.

Rodkin and Hodges (2003) review evidence indicating that although bullies do affiliate with each other, they are not exclusively segregated or isolated from their nonaggressive peers. They argue that if heterogeneous playground groupings of peers contain substantial numbers of aggressive, socially manipulative bullies, these groups may have the power to change playground norms regarding peer harassment—particularly so when high-status peers legitimize bullying via their approval or acceptance of it. These researchers note that children in low-status groups often suffer degradation, social exclusion, rejection, and ostracism. Membership in these groups will likely increase the chances that a child will be victimized by bullies and harassers.

Since bullying and harassment begin and end with the peer group, understanding the dynamics of peer-group relations on the playground is an essential prerequisite for addressing this problem. Studies of how children perceive their "enemies" have shown that hostility and simmering enmities among peers can often escalate into bullying and serious harassment (Rodkin & Hodges, 2003). A knowledge of these conflicts is essential to improve the social climate of the playground as well as the overall school (Leff et al., 2003). Focus groups, interviews, informant ratings, behavioral observations, and sociometric methods are tools that can and should be used to decode and understand the social tapestry of the peer group.

Classroom Settings and the Teacher

Although teachers are the most powerful influence within the classroom, they typically have little knowledge of, or influence with, peer-group dynamics and social relations that play out in other school settings. As a rule, they do not become involved in resolving peer-group conflicts—particularly on the playground. Serious peer conflicts are usually addressed by the school psychologist or counselor, with parental and teacher involvement regarded as ancillary.

However, classroom ecology can influence the extent to which the level of aggression exists among peers. For example, Henry et al. (2000) found that fourth-grade children who came from third-grade classrooms where the norms supported aggression showed elevated levels of aggression. In a now-classic longitudinal study, Kellam and his colleagues assessed the level of aggression in first-grade classrooms and used it to predict the aggressiveness of at-risk children through middle school (see Kellam, Ling, Merisca, Brown, & Ialongo, 1998). They found that students from high-aggressive first-grade classrooms were substantially more aggressive, years later in middle school, than matched control students in classrooms with low levels of aggression.

Given these findings, it is very important that teachers work closely with personnel from related services to address problems of aggression—particularly among primary-grade-level children. Teachers who ignore peer-related aggressive behavior may actually provide a pathway, albeit inadvertently, to peer victimization through aggression expressed as bullying. Another distressing finding is that teachers typically intervene in only about one-third of the peer harassment situations that come to their attention (Rodkin & Hodges, 2003; Rigby, 2001). Thus, by failing to take ownership of peer-related aggression in their classrooms, teachers may set the stage for higher levels of aggression in future years.

In our work with aggressive children, we find that they often do not take ownership or responsibility for the problems they cause others; instead, they present themselves as victims and tend to expect others to solve the problems they create. The following true vignette illustrates this point. It occurred several years ago and involved a

Colorado school psychologist named Billie S. Billie served three small elementary schools and was on a first-name basis with a third-grade girl in one of her schools, Sarah, who was a master of relational aggression. Sarah was smart, socially competent, highly manipulative, and quite skilled at getting other kids in trouble while proclaiming her own innocence. One day when Billie showed up at Sarah's school, the counselor and vice-principal were waiting at the door to tell her the latest things Sarah had done on the playground. They requested that she call Sarah in and deal with the situation. Billie arranged to meet with Sarah, and the following exchange occurred:

BILLIE: Sarah, I hear you've been having problems on the playground again!

SARAH: (*Looks at Billie; says nothing.*)

BILLIE: (*Attempting to engage Sarah in a problem-solving dialogue*) Sarah, what do you think people will say about your behavior on the playground?

SARAH: (*Thinking a minute, then looking at Billie*) Well, Billie, *some* people might say, you're not doing your job!

Increasingly, teachers are being asked to participate in prevention programs on aggression, violence, and bullying that teach students values and skills that are incompatible with aggression. Furthermore, positive behavior support interventions promote and reinforce positive values of respectfulness and self-responsibility. The teacher's modeling and teaching of such values can do a great deal to establish a classroom ecology that provides a counterforce to peer-related aggression and that will contribute to a positive classroom climate.

Teachers can also provide an important service to children and parents by supporting and protecting those students who appear vulnerable to peer-related aggression, bullying, and harassment. Teachers are in a solid position to screen and identify young aggressive students (i.e., primary grade level) whose aggression is directed mainly against peers and who may develop into full-fledged bullies and peer harassers. Form 6.1 in Chapter 6 contains a listing of behavioral characteristics that we have found to be highly effective in discriminating between such students and their normal peers. These behaviors can easily be converted into a frequency-based Likert scale for use by teachers and playground supervisors in screening/identifying such students.

IDENTIFYING BULLIES AND THEIR VICTIMS WITHIN THE CONTEXT OF SCHOOLING

Bullies and their victims are best known to and by the peer group where these social dynamics play out. The activities and roles of very obvious bullies and peer harassers may come to the attention of teachers and other adults in the school—particularly if their actions are egregious, repetitive, highly aggressive, and salient. However, the playground, during unstructured recess periods, affords perhaps the best opportunities to monitor peer-harassment dynamics and to identify chronic bullies and their victims. Teachers have some idea of the behavioral and psychosocial characteristics of bullies and their victims, but they often spend little time on the playground during recess periods. Although teachers possess extensive and usually accurate information about the behavioral characteristics of at-risk students with whom they are familiar, their lack of access to free play settings can prevent them from using their knowledge effectively in the detection and prevention of peer victimization. In contrast, playground supervisors, who are often paraprofessionals, have an excellent vantage point for detecting peer conflicts that often include harassment. Although they can be trained to monitor and detect instances of peer harassment, they generally only respond to and report the most obvious cases. As a rule, they are not instructed to look for and report peer-related abuse to school officials. Most acts of bullying and harassment are covert in nature, occur infrequently or sporadically, and tend to be perpetrated in settings and contexts that are not monitored effectively by adults.

Within the school setting, the key informants regarding bullying and victimization are peers, bullies and harassers, and their victims. Classroom teachers and playground supervisors are occasionally a rich source of information in this area as well. Parents can also be a useful, adjunctive information source, particularly if their child is a chronic victim of bullying. If we are to move from a largely reactive posture toward bullying and harassment, wherein only the most egregious cases are addressed by the school, to a proactive prevention strategy, we will need to involve peers, teachers, parents, and playground supervisors as key participants in the solution. Chapter 5 presents information on principles and recommended best practices in developing solutions to bullying and other forms of peer harassment.

Espelage and Swearer (2003) have reviewed the common methods used for assessing bullying and harassment in school settings: self-report, peer nominations, teacher nominations, and behavioral observations. As a rule, bullies are well known to peer-based informant groups and can be relatively easily identified; as noted earlier, their victims are more difficult to detect accurately, unless their victimization is chronic in nature. Estimates of the awareness of bullying and harassment among peers consistently approaches 70%. Peer nominations and self-reports of bullying are generally regarded by researchers as more accurate and valid than the judgments and nominations of teachers (Juvonen & Graham, 2001). Peer concurrence about who is frequently victimized and who does the victimizing is a powerful information source that needs to be considered carefully. Similarly, if certain students consistently identify themselves as victims of peer harassment, then such is probably the case—although some researchers argue that, when asked, victims may exaggerate the extent of their harassment.

The behavioral observation methods used to assess bullying within free play settings have a number of limitations and disadvantages. They involve socially intrusive measures that assess a large number of stimuli present in unstructured settings such as playgrounds. Furthermore, sampling becomes a serious issue with in vivo behavioral observations; as a rule, far fewer occasions are sampled than is necessary to adequately characterize a child or group's behavior. Bullying and peer victimization represent critical behavioral events that have a relatively low, and unpredictable, base rate of occurrence. Using in vivo behavioral observation methods to assess bullying and peer victimization on the playground is much like scanning the skies at night to detect satellites—the objects being sought come into view very infrequently and are difficult to detect when they do appear. Behavioral observations are best suited for recording relatively high-frequency forms of behavior.

In surveys of bullying, students typically are asked to indicate the extent to which they are aware of, have observed, and/or have been involved in bullying and peer harassment episodes. These survey responses are then tabulated and used to evaluate, in combination with interview responses, the extent to which bullying is a problem in a particular school. The surveys can also be used as pre- and postmeasures of bullying intervention programs. However, they are not useful for identifying the chronic bully or the chronic victim.

Orpinas, Horne, and Staniszewski (2003) reported the successful use of a Likert-type rating scale for assessing aggression and victimization in a study of bullying prevention with elementary-age students. The scale was developed originally for middle school students but has been successfully adapted for use in the elementary grades. The aggression subscale has 11 items and the victimization subscale has 10 items; both subscales demonstrate acceptable psychometric characteristics and require respondents to make frequency estimates of the extent to which they engage in aggressive/bullying types of behavior as well as how often they are victims of such behavior. In addition, both subscales proved to be sensitive measures of a year-long universal intervention program developed and implemented by Orpinas et al. (2003) to reduce bullying and victimization. A self-report Likert rating scale of this type is recommended for the following assessment tasks: (1) surveying school settings to determine the extent and seriousness of bullying and victimization, (2) the identification of chronic victimizers and victims, and (3) assessing the impact of schoolwide interventions to reduce bullying.

To solve a school's problems with bullying and peer harassment, it is important to identify both harassers and their victims. Pellegrini (2001) has extensively researched issues associated with these tasks and notes that the Olweus Bully/Victim Questionnaires for Children and Young Adolescents are the most frequently used self-report surveys in studies of bullying and victimization (see Olweus, 1992). These surveys can be used in either confidential or nonconfidential formats (i.e., students identify themselves on the questionnaire). Students are asked a series of questions as to the nature of their experiences in being victimized and in bullying others (e.g., "Have you been bullied by one or more students?" "How often have you been bullied?" and so on). Although self-reports are subject to bias and both under- and overreporting of incidents and their severity, they are still a valuable piece of the puzzle in determining the nature and extent of peer harassment problems in today's schools (see Pellegrini, 2001).

The perceptions of peers are an extremely valuable informational source in assessing the extent of peer harassment in schools and identifying both victims and perpetrators of bullying. Classroom rosters and peer nomination forms have been used successfully by Perry and his colleagues to validate who is victimized and who victimizes others among peer groups (Perry, Kusel, & Perry, 1988; Perry et al., 2001). Pellegrini and Bartini (2000) have successfully used this approach in their work on screening and identification as well. In this procedure, class rosters are provided to all students and a series of descriptive statements are read (e.g., "This child gets picked on a lot," "This child is mean to others," and so forth). Students then nominate or check the names of those peers whom they think represent or match the descriptive statements. A high level of convergence among peers regarding these descriptive statements provides powerful evidence for use in detecting and treating the problems of school bullying. Investigators should also look for convergence between the self-reports of victims and the peer nominations regarding victimization and harassment.

Bullies are likely to emerge out of the pool of highly aggressive students who reside within the peer group. In a similar vein, potential victims are likely to be contained in groups of peers who are socially unskilled, withdrawing, easily intimidated, neglected, and excluded from peer-controlled activities. Membership in such groups increases the likelihood of victimization, just as membership in a deviant and aggressive peer group increases the likelihood that its members will bully others.

Chapter 6 discusses the proactive early screening and identification of preschool and elementary-age students who are having either externalizing and/or internalizing behavior problems in school. A complete screening and identification system is described and illustrated for this purpose (Walker & Severson, 1990; Walker et al., 1995). This system can be implemented on a schoolwide basis to screen students for these problems. Those who emerge through its three screening gates are likely to have very serious behavior problems of either an externalizing or internalizing nature. Using self reports and peer-teacher nominations, as appropriate and feasible, these identified students should be further assessed for their status as bullies and/or victims. We would expect to find bullies and provocative victims among the pool of identified externalizers, and passive/submissive victims among the pool of identified internalizers.

The screening and identification of school bullies and their victims is a high-stakes and controversial process and should involve multiple methods and sources of information to reduce the likelihood of error. Relying on only one method or informational source in this regard is ill advised due to the risks associated with false positives and false negatives. In this context, schools are most vulnerable to parental pressures mounted by the caregivers of both identified bullies and their victims. Research strongly suggests that a combination of self-report, peer nomination, observational, and informant ratings be used when (1) determining the extent of bullying and peer harassment within a school, and (2) identifying the frequent harassers and their chronic victims (Espelage & Swearer, 2003). When these measures are confirmatory of each other, then confidence in the assessment outcomes should increase proportionately.

CONCLUSION

This chapter has described the current landscape of bullying and peer-based harassment in today's schools. The research evidence indicates that this phenomenon has multiple determinants and is subject to a diverse range of risk factors and exacerbating conditions. Because of their social impact and capacity for producing destructive outcomes, bullying and harassing behaviors have increased to a level that can no longer be ignored in the hope that they will resolve themselves without adult intervention and attention. Recent court decisions and legislation have clearly established harassment and bullying in schools as unacceptable and/or illegal acts that can no longer be ignored.

Much has been learned over the past decade about how to buffer, ameliorate, and prevent peer harassment in the schooling context. Effective interventions require attention to the school environment as well as to victims and bullies. It is essential that solutions to this problem are "owned" by parents, bullies, victims, peers, and especially educators and related services personnel within the school. Chapter 5 discusses best practices and proven strategies that target peer-based harassment.

5

Solutions for Bullying and Peer Harassment in the School Setting

with STEPHEN G. SMITH

Chapter 4 provided extensive documentation of the causes, dynamics, and extent of bullying and peer-based harassment in school settings as well as the influences that appear to shape and sustain the bully and victim roles among certain youth. Recommended approaches were described for assessing bullying and harassment, with the goal of detecting bullies and victims and designing interventions for them. This chapter focuses on strategies for preventing, ameliorating, and remediating these growing problems in our schools. Considerations for school personnel responsible for addressing bullying and harassment are discussed along with descriptions of recommended intervention strategies.

KEY CONSIDERATIONS REGARDING EFFECTIVE SCHOOL-BASED EFFORTS TO INTERVENE WITH BULLYING AND HARASSMENT

School districts and school staffs face complex, and often unfamiliar, challenges when attempting to intervene effectively with bullying and harassing students. The often covert nature of these events makes them difficult to detect, and our relatively limited ability to observe and analyze them, when they do occur, makes the design and implementation of effective interventions somewhat problematic.

There are myriad social constraints and considerations that impact our screening, identification, and intervention efforts. For instance, many students are characteristically reluctant to speak out or seek adult help in these types of situations. Similarly, teachers, other school staff, and parents may be reluctant, unwilling, or unable to initiate and pursue the actions necessary to intervene with students who display bullying and harassing behaviors. School personnel may find that parents are defensive and reluctant or unwilling to address the child's problem behavior, whether that of perpetration or victimization. Parents often find that school personnel are subject to similar limitations, although they are largely self-imposed.

In addition, the current social climate within schools places considerable stigma on youth who are accused of engaging in harassment of any kind. Furthermore, the determination of our society to view harassment (including harassment associated with bullying) as a criminal and civil offense, with the attendant legal ramifications, attaches a substantial accountability factor to the actions taken by those school officials responsible for today's students. The district, school, and/or individual staff member may incur substantial legal liability and financial risk, both institutionally and on a personal level, if found negligent in cases involving harassment of any type. Interventions for bullying and harassment can also be quite difficult, complex, and costly, depending on the nature and severity of the problem. Many educators do not view such interventions as cost effective or worth the effort, particularly given that peer harassment and bullying traditionally have been regarded as peer-owned problems, to be worked out within the peer group in the absence of adult involvement. Recent court cases, however, have now rendered this option moot. The risks of not doing something about serious bullying and peer harassment currently outweigh the risks involved in formally addressing these problems.

Addressing the perpetrator's behavior, however, is only half of the task. Ongoing victim intervention and support must be part of any effective and lasting solution (Smith & Sprague, 2003). In fact, effective intervention in a bullying/harassment dynamic should address the specific needs of a variety of impacted individuals that includes the victim, the perpetrator, parents, school staff, peers, and others negatively affected by the problem behavior. A comprehensive and effective bullying intervention, initiated in response to ongoing, widespread, and/or pervasive bullying and harassment, may well stress school and district financial resources. This sort of demand on a school's resources should be built into its financial planning in the same manner as are the costs of school safety and academic reform measures.

Reactionary (i.e., after the fact) interventions that have a crisis ambience to them are potentially the most costly. They are the least likely to be effective and are difficult to implement successfully, because they usually involve making changes in an established and long-held set of practices. These interventions typically are punishment based and are focused on one or two individuals: the perpetrator(s), perhaps the victim(s), and occasionally, selected bystanders. Proactive or prevention interventions, aimed at addressing bullying through education (e.g., social skills training) and providing positive behavioral interventions and supports, are typically less expensive to implement, are generally acceptable to most school personnel (particularly if they are universal in nature), and are less socially stigmatizing (Orpinas, Horne, & Staniszewski, 2003). These interventions (1) can be used to address a wide range of problem behavior in addition to bullying and harassment, (2) are usually focused on *all* students in the school, and (3) are based on proven principles of teaching, reinforcing, and recognizing positive, expected forms of behavior (e.g., empathy, respect, positive regard for others, and responsibility).

A consensus of research (Wolery, Bailey, & Sugai, 1988; Olweus, 1991, 1994, 1996; Walker, Ramsey, & Gresham, 2004; Snell, MacKenzie, & Frey, 2002) suggests that interventions aimed at bully/victim problems should be the product of a coordinated and cooperative effort involving all concerned parties in every target environment and at every level (i.e., playground, schoolwide, family, and individual) in order to be effective. We recognize that although professional interventions and supports at the family level are difficult to implement consistently, every effort should be made to involve parents as intervention participants to the extent they are willing and capable of such involvement in them.

The school environment provides the only relatively accessible setting for the consistent implementation of interventions and services targeting bully/victim behaviors. Olweus (1996) supports the creation of a caring, positive school environment as a first step for intervening in the bully/victim cycle. The creation and maintenance of such an environment is well within the capacity of most schools. There is some indication that the provision of consistent and universal (i.e., all students and staff) training in appropriate responses to bully/victim situations can help eliminate a great deal of this problem behavior (Grossman et al., 1997). Whole-school interventions of this sort can target early problem behaviors such as teasing before they accelerate and lead to more extreme problems involving bullying and serious harassment. Schools need to develop and consistently apply rules that prohibit bullying and hold regular class booster meetings to provide repeated exposure to those rules (Olweus, 1996; Orpinas et al., 2003). One basic and proven method for establishing a bullying- and harassment-free school climate is to ask all students to sign a pledge to not tease, harass, bully, intimidate, or put down others. Reports from schools that have tried this simple approach indicate that it makes a positive difference in the number of incidents that occur on school grounds (see Chapter 4; see also Olweus, 1994, 1996).

RECOMMENDED STEPS AND MODEL PROGRAMS FOR USE BY SCHOOLS IN ADDRESSING BULLYING AND PEER HARASSMENT

Recommended Steps

Overall, schools seeking to reduce or eliminate bullying and harassment problems should follow a series of steps designed to introduce, teach, imbed, and infuse a systems-wide operational intervention program that is ongoing, supported at district and school administrative levels, is research based, financially feasible, and acceptable to the various stakeholders involved. These steps should include the following:

1. Formulate and implement an anti-bullying and anti-harassment policy at the school campus or district levels.
2. Assess the nature and extent of the problem.
3. Select an appropriate schoolwide response.
4. Solicit family support.
5. Train all staff, students, and families.
6. Promote active supervision of students in common areas.
7. Respond to chronic bullies with increasing supports, sanctions, and proven interventions.
8. Assist chronic victims to be more assertive, gain friendship skills, and avoid dangerous situations.
9. Record all instances of bullying behavior and change your approach according to emerging patterns.

Environmental manipulations and rearrangements are examples of preventing bullying and harassment through environmental design. They are simple and easy to make—costing, as a rule, very little in the way of fiscal resources—and they can effectively reduce the undesired behaviors of bullies. Research by Olweus (1994) indicates that the number of students reporting victimization begins to drop off, over time, as students advance through the grade levels. Two main reasons are offered for this outcome as follows: (1) As students age, they generally become less vulnerable to intimidating and other antisocial behaviors associated with bullying and harassment; they develop both prosocial and anti-bullying strategies (often called coping skills), and (2) As students progress through grade levels, the perceived imbalance of power (one of the characteristics associated with bullying) between perpetrator and victim may be reduced due to one or more factors, including (a) a reduced number of students who are older and therefore fewer opportunities for interaction with students in which age and social standing may be the enabling factors; (b) decreases in physical differences within and between grade level peers; and (c) increasing development of stable, ongoing friendships or inclusion in socially supportive peer subgroups.

These findings suggest an intervention that involves simple environmental manipulations and rearrangements designed to isolate younger from older students by grade level as much as possible—specifically targeting recess, lunch, and other relatively unstructured or lightly supervised periods. These arrangements can be accomplished by scheduling grade-level recess and transition periods at staggered intervals and by maintaining separate, physically isolated lunch, play, and free-time areas for each grade level.

Clinical research (Sprague & Walker, 2000; Lewis, Sugai, & Colvin, 1998; Grossman et al., 1997) indicates that universal, proactive, and schoolwide behavior support programs, in conjunction with behavior-specific supports for at-risk students, can be effective with all but 5–10% of the students in most of today's schools. These 5–10% usually have severe behavior disorders and are moderately to extremely antisocial. Their behavior disorders are often resistant to treatment due to complex environmental risk factors external to the school setting. Members of this small group of students require individually tailored interventions in order to effectively address their problem behavior. Chronic bullies frequently fall into this 5–10% of students.

Positive behavior support approaches that rely primarily on universal, schoolwide interventions have become very popular with educators and are being adopted by school staffs on a broad scale nationally (Sugai & Horner, 2002). Such approaches are quite effective in creating positive school climates and in involving a majority of school staff in implementing the interventions. Typically, they net dramatic effects in reducing disciplinary referrals to the principal's office by teachers. Very few of these efforts, however, have been applied to the problems of school bullying and peer harassment, even though they could potentially impact these harmful behaviors. We recommend that any universal, schoolwide approach implemented to address problem behavior also target bullying and harassment. In addition, it is essential that measures of bullying and harassment (e.g., self-reports, student and staff surveys, focus groups, etc.) also be used, along with other outcome measures, to document intervention effects.

Model Programs That Address Peer Bullying and Harassment

This section describes programs known to be effective in addressing bullying and harassment problems. Interventions include (1) a model schoolwide intervention combining positive behavior support (PBS) principles and bullying prevention procedures; (2) the Olweus Bullying Intervention Program; (3) the School-Wide Positive Behavior Support (SWPBS) intervention model; (4) the active supervision of common areas; (5) the Second Step Violence Prevention Curriculum; (6) Steps to respect: A bullying prevention program; and (7) Bully-proofing your school: A comprehensive approach for elementary schools.

Combining Positive Behavior Support Practices and Bullying Prevention Procedures

Orpinas et al. (2003) recently reported on a bullying prevention program, implemented over a 1-year period in a single elementary school, that combined the principles and procedures of PBS approaches with the procedures developed by Olweus (1993). The intervention was universal in nature, involved nearly 600 elementary students in K–5 grades and 24 teachers as participants, and was based on a collaboration model. Designed to reduce aggression and victimization by changing the school environment, this intervention illustrates important techniques and necessary steps for consideration by school personnel concerned with solving the problem of bullying and victimization.

Orpinas et al. (2003) began their intervention by establishing a schoolwide committee, composed of one teacher per grade level, paraprofessionals, a parent, the school counselor and the principal, that met monthly during the school year. The charge of the committee was to assume the leadership role in implementing a comprehensive plan for improving the school's climate, teaching social skills, and preventing bullying. A series of focus groups was held with students to gauge their perceptions of the school's problems with verbal and physical aggression as well as the school's policies. Students were also engaged in the problem-solving process through their completion of the aggression/victimization subscales.

The survey results and student feedback were analyzed, as were teacher recommendations, and used to carefully tailor the intervention components needed to address the specific problems the school was experiencing. The school's staff, in conjunction with the leadership committee, decided on three delivery strategies for solving the school's problems: (1) change school norms and policies so as to create a positive school climate; (2) educate and train students; and (3) provide staff development training in implementation. The following techniques were applied over the school year in support of these goals:

1. Five core values were developed and taught throughout the school year (be respectful, responsible, honest, ready to learn, and be your personal best).
2. To support achievement of each core value, school and classroom rules were developed that discouraged teasing, name calling, and put-downs, and signs were posted throughout the school.
3. The student conduct code was rewritten to incorporate these core values and rules and renamed *The Handbook for Success*.
4. All students were trained in the Peace-Able Place Program (a.k.a. the Too Good for Violence program) that teaches conflict-resolution skills and strategies, anger management, respect for self and others, and effective communication. (Teachers and the school counselor jointly taught these lessons.)
5. All teachers completed a 20-hour training program on comprehensive schoolwide strategies for bullying and aggression prevention, including conflict-resolution strategies, character education, and behavior management.
6. In collaboration with experts, the school staff created a bullying prevention plan that was implemented throughout the school year.
7. Teachers and other school staff recognized and positively reinforced students when they observed them displaying the core values and supporting the rules.

This intervention produced statistically significant reductions in aggression and victimization for students in grades K–2; students in grades 3–5 showed significant changes on self-reported rates of victimization but not aggression. This intervention was impressive in how it was designed, planned, and implemented. The full engagement of students and teachers in the intervention was viewed by the researchers as a key to its success.

The Olweus Bullying Intervention Program

The Olweus school-based bullying intervention program is based on principles that create school environments characterized by warmth, positive social interest, adult involvement, firm limits, clearly defined standards governing acceptable and unacceptable behavior, and consistent noncorporal consequences for bullying and harassment behaviors. The Olweus program requires the following actions by schools:

- Staff take responsibility for reducing or eliminating bullying behavior.
- Staff develop and promote clear moral and ethical positions against bullying.
- Staff develop and set long- and short-term goals that target the entire school population through the implementation of systems-based and individually oriented intervention strategies.
- The program is established as a consistent and stable component of the school environment.
- Staff promote and maintain a positive school climate that encompasses all students.
- Parents are involved, as feasible, in the intervention program.

As prerequisites, this program calls for staff and parents to be aware of their school's bullying and harassment problems, and that staff and parents commit to reducing or eliminating them. The awareness component is accomplished through the collection and analysis of data (questionnaires and surveys). Committed involvement is accomplished through collecting and sharing information and agreeing to work toward solutions.

The Olweus program implements intervention procedures at schoolwide, classroom, and individual levels:

Schoolwide interventions are intended to positively influence the entire student body (Sugai & Horner, 1994; Sprague, Walker, Golly, et al., 2001) and are designed to reduce or eliminate bullying by improving school climate, culture, and instructional programs (Grossman et al., 1997). These schoolwide measures include:

- Assessment of the problem through surveys and questionnaires
- Convening of school conferences on bully/victim issues with staff, students, and parents
- Increased adult supervision in unstructured, high-census common areas (e.g., playgrounds, cafeterias)

- Improvement in common area infrastructures (e.g., more attractive playground equipment)
- Problem-solving efforts with staff, students, and parents
- Establishment of a school-based prosocial improvement team dedicated to school culture and climate issues

Classroom activities involve the establishment of behavioral expectations, rules, and positive and negative consequences in addition to the implementation of instructional programs and activities. These interventions include:

- Creating school rules prohibiting bullying
- Establishing positive reinforcement (praise) for appropriate behavior
- Establishing negative consequences for inappropriate behavior
- Conducting role playing, cooperative learning groups, and positive classroom activities
- Regularly scheduled class meetings devoted to solving the problem of bullying
- Meetings with teacher, students, and parents

Individual activities are intended to change the behavior of individual students. Individual interventions target both the bully and the victim—and, less often, those peers collaterally involved in bully/victim interactions. Recommended individual intervention activities include:

- Immediate and ongoing one-on-one talks of a serious nature with both bully and victim
- Separate, ongoing debriefings with the participating students and their parents
- Joint talks between the bully and his or her parents and the victim and his or her parents (includes the school psychologist and/or counselor, whenever possible)
- Provision of social and behavioral support resources for parents of participants
- Discussion groups for parents of perpetrators
- Change in placement of bully/victim (classroom, school, etc.), as required

The Olweus program has been shown to be successful across a wide range of schools and diverse populations in several countries. Reductions of 50% or more in bully/victim problems have been obtained in studies of the program in Norway, where it was developed. These reductions have been replicated numerous times in a variety of school settings and include (1) collateral effects such as a reduction in general anti-social behavior (e.g., vandalism, fighting, theft, substance abuse, truancy), (2) improvement in social climate and school culture, (3) reduction of target behaviors in nonschool community settings, and (4) an increase in student attachment to school. The Olweus bullying intervention is included among the 11 blueprint programs for violence prevention published by the Center for the Study and Prevention of Violence, Institute of Behavioral Science, at the University of Colorado at Boulder

The School-Wide Positive Behavior Support Intervention Model

The SWPBS model is a proactive prevention approach focused on supporting the behavior of all students across all grades and school settings (see Chapters 2 and 3). It is designed to increase the capacity of schools to develop, institute, and sustain comprehensive behavior support systems at schoolwide, classroom, nonclassroom, and individual student levels.

SWPBS incorporates research-validated development and support activities in several critical areas:

- Development and ongoing administrative support of a school-based PBS team
- Development and dissemination of clear schoolwide behavioral expectations
- Procedures for establishing and teaching schoolwide rules based on the school's behavioral expectations
- Procedures for teaching appropriate prosocial skills
- Systematic prompting for appropriate behavior
- Development, dissemination, and consistent use of schoolwide rewards for appropriate, expected behavior
- Development, dissemination, and consistent use of schoolwide consequences for inappropriate, problem behavior
- Procedures for establishing and maintaining the ongoing monitoring and record keeping of student behavior
- Development and implementation of increased behavioral supports for at-risk and high-risk students

Research on SWPBS model programs has reported an average 42% decrease in student behavior problems (as measured by office discipline referrals; Sugai & Horner, 1994; Taylor-Green et al., 1997) in the first year of implementation, with additional reductions noted in subsequent years. Chapter 3 provides a comprehensive description of this approach, including a self-assessment and recommended staff development procedures.

Active Supervision

The approach of active supervision (Smith & Sprague, 2001) is based on the following key principles (Colvin, Sugai, Good, & Lee, 1997):

- The provision of proactive, positive behavior supports
- The consistent application of nonhostile, nonphysical consequences

- Monitoring and surveillance of activities inside and outside the school
- Adult authority in response to bullying and harassment
- Application of a team-based approach

WHAT IS ACTIVE SUPERVISION?

Active supervision is a term applied to a multiple-component method of providing student behavior support and management (Smith & Sprague, 2001). Active supervision methods work well in settings that share the following characteristics: (1) large area, (2) high census (i.e., many students), (3) lightly staffed (i.e., one or two adults for every 80+ kids), and (4) unstructured (student-directed) activities in areas such as playgrounds, cafeterias, hallways, etc.

HOW DOES ACTIVE SUPERVISION WORK?

Active supervision works by supporting appropriate student behavior, giving supervisors increased opportunities for providing high rates of positive contact with a large percentage of the available students, giving supervisors increased opportunities for correcting inappropriate student behavior, and providing supervisors with effective methods of reinforcing appropriate behavior and sanctions and consequences for inappropriate behaviors. Our experience with this method has shown that high rates of positive contact with individuals or groups of students can substantially reduce student problem behavior.

THE ELEMENTS OF ACTIVE SUPERVISION

There are two primarily physical elements to active supervision: movement and scanning. *Effective movement techniques* should (1) be constant, (2) randomized, (3) target known problem areas, activities, groups, and individuals, and (4) increase opportunities for close, proximal contact with problem areas, activities, groups, and individuals.

Instituting effective movement techniques requires (1) frequent or constant rates of movement within the area to be supervised; (2) randomized, unpredictable patterns of movement; and (3) movement calculated to target known problem areas with regularity, and to bring the supervisor into close proximity to problem activities, groups, or individuals. Examples of constant and/or randomized movement are:

- The supervisor moves an average of 30 feet per minute while supervising playground activities.
- The supervisor covers six different activity areas during recess, making close contact with each one at least two times during a 15-minute recess.

- The supervisor varies the order of contact in the different activity areas: on first pass areas *a, b, c, d, e,* and *f* are covered; next pass would cover areas *c, e, a, f, d,* and then *b.*

Two examples of targeting known problem areas, activities, groups, and individuals follow:

- The supervisor knows (from past experience and observation) that there is typically a great deal of arguing during recess at the fifth-grade tetherball game. The supervisor begins each fifth-grade recess at the tetherball area, greets students as they come out, and restates rules and expected behaviors.
- The supervisor suspects that a loosely affiliated group of four to six problem students seems to get into trouble with peers and supervisors nearly every recess. The supervisor makes sure to schedule several randomly spaced close-proximity contacts with this group during each recess.

Effective scanning techniques in common areas include (1) targeting both appropriate and inappropriate behavior, (2) targeting known problem areas, activities, groups, and individuals, and (3) using both visual and aural cues. Common area supervisors should constantly shift visual and aural attention to cover all areas under their purview and target both appropriate and inappropriate behavior. Utilizing both visual and aural scanning methods extends the adult's ability to supervise large areas and increases opportunities for positive contact.

There are two positive behavior support components to active supervision: positive contact and positive reinforcement. *Positive contact* consists of (1) using a friendly, helpful, and open demeanor when interacting with students; (2) establishing and maintaining a proactive approach that reinforces expected, appropriate student behavior and also prompts noncontingent positive adult attention; and (3) maintaining high rates of both specific and noncontingent positive contacts with all students.

Positive contacts with students during movement and scanning activities should be preventive in nature, with supervisors engaging students, in groups and individually, on a fairly constant basis. Positive contact should be initiated with any student based solely on the absence of inappropriate behavior. The delivery of positive contacts by supervisors should also be noncontingent, meaning that, from time to time, students receive praise for simply being themselves.

The second behavioral tool necessary for effective active supervision, *positive reinforcement*, requires the delivery of reinforcement (i.e., behavior-specific praise) to groups or individuals when they engage in appropriate and expected forms of behavior.

The Second Step Violence Prevention Curriculum

The Second Step Violence Prevention Curriculum, developed by the Committee for Children in Seattle, is one of the best approaches available for creating a positive peer culture of caring and civility, as well as for teaching specific strategies for controlling/managing anger and resolving conflicts without resorting to bullying/harassment, coercion, or violence. This curriculum was recently rated, by an expert panel of the Safe and Drug Free Schools, Division of the U.S. Department of Education, as *the* most effective of all those currently available for creating safe and positive schools.

Second Step is a promising, multicomponent curricular intervention that provides systematic instruction in interpersonal skills such as empathy, anger management, impulse control, and conflict resolution, which can be used in both traditional and alternative educational settings. Grossman et al. (1997) used six matched pairs of urban and suburban elementary schools and randomly assigned them to intervention or comparison conditions to assess the program's effectiveness. Students in the intervention group were taught the Second Step curriculum two to three times per week over a 12-week period. Using a structured protocol, trained observers (blind as to condition) found that in unstructured school settings (e.g., playground, cafeteria), students in the intervention group showed decreased physically aggressive behavior and increased neutral and prosocial behaviors ($p < .05$). The gains for the experimental group of students were significantly greater than for controls. A 3-year longitudinal evaluation study of this program is currently underway, and a number of pilot studies are highly encouraging.

Steps to Respect

The Steps to Respect Bullying Prevention Curriculum incorporates research-based principles and instructional activities that foster academic skills, build social–emotional competence, and teach positive social values. The curriculum integrates academic skills (e.g., oral expression, written composition, analytic reasoning skills, vocabulary enrichment, literary analysis, reading comprehension) with core social–emotional competencies (e.g., self-management, social skills, perspective taking and empathy, communication skills, emotional management, risk-assessment and decision-making skills, setting and achieving positive goals, conflict resolution, friendship building). In addition to the student curricular elements, Steps to Respect has whole-staff and parent components designed to augment and support the instructional units (see Figure 5.1).

Steps to Respect is intended to be used over 3–4 years, with Part 1 designed for third- to fourth-grade students, Part 2 geared toward fourth- to fifth-grade students, and Part 3 used with fifth- to sixth-grade students. The program, curriculum, and instructional activities are designed for schoolwide implementation, with the teaching staff ideally providing the instructional pieces and the staff as a whole supporting the behavioral intervention by taking reports and acting as coaches. Recent research indicates that programs similar to Steps to Respect in form and content (in this case, the Second Step Violence Prevention Curriculum), when used in conjunction with a schoolwide positive behavior support program such as Best Behavior (see Chapter 3), can be very effective in reducing the incidence and severity of many behavior prob-

Student Components	Skill Units
	• Identification of bullying and peer harassment
	• Identification of racism, sexual prejudice, sexual harassment
	Literature Units
	• Two literature units per level
	• Language arts objectives tied to social–emotional objectives
	• Activities tied to various content areas (geography, history, art, etc.)
Teacher and Staff Components	All staff trained to receive and effectively respond to student reports of bullying and harassment (includes volunteers, bus and cafeteria personnel, office staff, etc.)
	• Learn and practice specific skills for responding to reports
	• Learn and practice specific skills for coaching students involved in bullying incidents, both perpetrators and victims
	• Learn to use a common language and tie activities to the curriculum
Administrator Components	Leadership role in implementation
	• Secures commitment from staff and parents
	• Develops school anti-bullying policy, disciplinary and reporting activities
	• Provides for staff training
	• Provides for parent information and supports
	• Monitors the program
Parent/Family Components	Provision of information regarding program, expectations, consequences, etc.
	• Invited to ongoing discussion and participation in program
	• 1.5-hour informational overview on program content and strategies
	• Take-home handouts for each skill unit

FIGURE 5.1. Components of the Steps to Respect Bullying Prevention Curriculum.

lems (Sprague & Golly, 2004). An ongoing 3-year study of this program is currently underway in Seattle area schools.

Bully-Proofing Your School

Bully-Proofing Your School (Garrity, Jens, Porter, Sager, & Short-Camilli, 1994) provides a comprehensive approach to the problem of bullying along with intervention guidelines, a schoolwide intervention program, staff training, student instruction, victim support components, perpetrator support curriculum, a parent/family component, and a resource guide with reproducible presentation and teaching materials. The program is geared for consumer-friendly teaching and implementation; the curriculum is flexible and designed to be completed in 2–3 months. Bully-Proofing enlists a school staff member (e.g., administrator, school counselor, school psychologist, behavior support specialist, teacher, social worker) to act in the role of facilitator. This facilitator takes the initiative in organizing and implementing the five main program components: staff training, student instruction, victim support, perpetrator interventions, and collaboration with parents and families. The intended outcomes of Bully-Proofing include increases in school attachment by students, student and staff perceptions of school safety, positive school culture and climate, and student skills relating to positive character development and personal and community responsibility.

LEGAL ISSUES CONCERNING BULLYING AND HARASSMENT IN SCHOOLS

It is strongly recommended that educators and others working with school children in this area become familiar with the laws and policies concerning bullying and harassment that are in effect in their local and state institutions. Table 5.1 presents selected state laws and policies considered to be of critical importance to effective legal and policy treatment of bullying and harassment problems. Table 5.2 provides the text for Oregon House Bill 3403, which was designed to address bullying and harassment in Oregon schools. This bill was passed by the Oregon State House of Representatives on May 17, 2001, and by the Oregon State Senate on May 30, 2001. It is considered to be one of the most comprehensive state legislative treatments of this problem to date. The bill requires the Superintendent of Public Instruction to develop model policies prohibiting harassment, intimidation, or bullying on school grounds, at school activities, on school transportation, or at school bus stops. It also requires each school district to adopt policies against harassment, intimidation, and bullying.

This legislative act mandates that every Oregon school district develop and implement anti-bullying, -intimidation, and -harassment policies. The act defines bullying, intimidation, and harassment in legal terms rather than leaving it to school districts or the state Office of Education, as recommended by Limber and Small (2003). Rules and guidelines for developing district policies are clearly stipulated. The act also calls for districts to develop and implement specific guarantees, protections, and consequences for responding to incidences of bullying and harassment. Other states have developed, or are in the process of developing, legislation similar in scope to the Oregon bill, which is considered model legislation in this area.

There is a growing national emphasis on, and legal requirements for, developing anti-bullying and harassment policies on both district- and school-specific levels (U.S. Department of Education/Office for Civil Rights and the National Association of Attorneys General, 1999). Currently, the development and dissemination of an anti-

TABLE 5.1. Features of State Anti-Bullying and Harassment Policy, Statute, and Law

	CO	MI	CA	OR	WA	OK	WV	NH	U.S. DOE*	NAAG*
Mandates "safe, secure, peaceful" school environment	Yes**	***	Yes		Yes	Yes	Yes	Yes		
Specifically mentions bullying?	Yes	Yes	Yes	Yes	Yes	Yes	Yes	Yes	Yes	
Specifically mentions harassment?		Yes	Yes	Yes	Yes	Yes	Yes	Yes		Yes
Specifically mentions intimidation?		Yes		Yes	Yes	Yes	Yes			
Specifically prohibits bullying, harassment, or intimidation?	Yes	Yes		Yes	Yes	Yes	Yes		N/A	
Bullying defined?	Yes	Yes		Yes	Yes	Yes	Yes	Yes		
Harassment defined?		Yes	Yes	Yes	Yes	Yes	Yes			Yes
Intimidation defined?		Yes		Yes	Yes	Yes	Yes			
School-site specific?		Yes	Yes			Yes				
Mandates a statewide policy?										
Mandates a county- or district-level policy?	Yes		Yes	Yes	Yes	Yes	Yes			
Mandates a school-by-school policy?		Yes	Yes					Yes		
Mandates oversight by representative panel, task force, team, etc.		Yes	Yes	Yes	Yes	Yes	Yes	Yes		
Mandates needs assessment						Yes		Yes		
Mandates policy training for staff		Yes			Yes		Yes	Yes		
Mandates clinical training for staff								Yes		
Mandates a school plan?			Yes					Yes		
Mandates investigative procedures?		Yes		Yes			Yes	Yes		
Mandates or outlines specific adult responses?				Yes			Yes	Yes		
Mandates anonymity for reporting students?		Yes		Yes			Yes	Yes		
Addresses reprisal, retaliation, or false accusation		Yes		Yes	Yes		Yes	Yes		
Sets out student consequences?	Yes	Yes		Yes			Yes			
Sets out adult responsibilities?				Yes	Yes		Yes	Yes		
Sets out conditions for school/employee indemnification or immunity?	Yes	Yes		Yes	Yes		Yes	Yes		
Critical behavioral elements/features of law, statute, rule, or policy										
Gestures	Yes	Yes				Yes				
Written	Yes	Yes			Yes	Yes	Yes			
Verbal	Yes	Yes		Yes	Yes	Yes	Yes	Yes		

(continued)

112

TABLE 5.1. (*continued*)

	CO	MI	CA	OR	WA	OK	WV	NH	U.S. DOE*	NAAG*
Physical	Yes	Yes			Yes	Yes	Yes	Yes	Yes	
Harm to student		Yes	Yes	Yes	Yes	Yes	Yes	Yes		
Harm to student's property		Yes	Yes	Yes	Yes	Yes				
Reasonable fear of harm to person or their property		Yes	Yes	Yes	Yes	Yes				
Based on race, ethnicity		Yes	Yes	Yes					Yes	Yes
Based on gender		Yes	Yes	Yes					Yes	Yes
Based on religion or creed		Yes		Yes					Yes	Yes
Based on sexual orientation		Yes		Yes					Yes	Yes
Based on disability or physical attributes		Yes		Yes					Yes	Yes
Based on socioecomic or other distinguishing features		Yes	Yes							
Disruption of education or educational mission by any of the above		Yes		Yes	Yes	Yes	Yes			

Note. The information in this table was collected from state and federal legislative and Department of Education websites. Searches of statute and constitutional law, as well as state and federal policy, were conducted to the greatest extent possible. The information presented is intended to illustrate an example of law and policy addressing bullying and harassment in schools and should not be regarded as a complete or comprehensive legal source, or the authors as legal experts.

* The U.S. Department of Education (U.S. DOE) and the National Association of Attorneys General (NAAG) are not rule- or policymaking bodies and, as such, cannot promulgate or enforce law or policy. In cases where the item indicates, "Mandates," the reader should substitute "Suggests" or "Recommends."

** A "Yes" response indicates that the documents available at the time of publication addressed the item in some form. Some items were more fully addressed by some state documents than by others.

*** A blank response indicates that the item was not addressed by the documents available at the time of publication.

TABLE 5.2. Oregon House Bill 3403

Section 1. The Legislative Assembly finds that:

(1) A safe and civil environment is necessary for students to learn and achieve high academic standards.

(2) Harassment, intimidation or bullying, like other disruptive or violent behavior, is conduct that disrupts a student's ability to learn and a school's ability to educate its students in a safe environment.

(3) Students learn by example. The legislature commends school administrators, faculty, staff and volunteers for demonstrating appropriate behavior, treating others with civility and respect and refusing to tolerate harassment, intimidation or bullying.

Section 2. As used in sections 1 to 7 of this 2001 Act, "harassment, intimidation or bullying" means any act that substantially interferes with a student's educational benefits, opportunities or performance, that takes place on or immediately adjacent to school grounds, at any school-sponsored activity, on school-provided transportation or at any official school bus stop, and that has the effect of:

(1) Physically harming a student or damaging a student's property;

(2) Knowingly placing a student in reasonable fear of physical harm to the student or damage to the student's property; or

(3) Creating a hostile educational environment.

Section 3. Each school district shall adopt a policy prohibiting harassment, intimidation or bullying. School districts are encouraged to develop the policy after consultation with parents and guardians, school employees, volunteers, students, administrators and community representatives.

(2) School districts are encouraged to include in the policy:

   (a) A statement prohibiting harassment, intimidation or bullying;

   (b) A definition of harassment, intimidation or bullying that is consistent with section 2 of this 2001 Act;

   (c) A description of the type of behavior expected from each student;

   (d) A statement of the consequences and appropriate remedial action for a person who commits an act of harassment, intimidation or bullying;

   (e) A procedure for reporting an act of harassment, intimidation or bullying, including a provision that permits a person to report an act of harassment, intimidation or bullying anonymously. Nothing in this paragraph may be construed to permit formal disciplinary action solely on the basis of an anonymous report;

   (f) A procedure for prompt investigation of a report of an act of harassment, intimidation or bullying;

   (g) A statement of the manner in which a school district will respond after an act of harassment, intimidation or bullying is reported, investigated and confirmed;

   (h) A statement of the consequences and appropriate remedial action for a person found to have committed an act of harassment, intimidation or bullying;

   (i) A statement prohibiting reprisal or retaliation against any person who reports an act of harassment, intimidation or bullying and stating the consequences and appropriate remedial action for a person who engages in such reprisal or retaliation;

(continued)

TABLE 5.2. (*continued*)

    (j) A statement of the consequences and appropriate remedial action for a person found to have falsely accused another of having committed an act of harassment, intimidation or bullying as a means of reprisal or retaliation or as a means of harassment, intimidation or bullying;

    (k) A statement of how the policy is to be publicized within the district, including a notice that the policy applies to behavior at school-sponsored activities; and

    (l) The identification by job title of school officials responsible for ensuring that policy is implemented.

Section 4. Each school district shall adopt a policy prohibiting harassment, intimidation or bullying and transmit a copy of the policy to the Superintendent of Public Instruction by January 1, 2004.

Section 5.

    (1) A school employee, student or volunteer may not engage in reprisal or retaliation against a victim of, witness to or person with reliable information about an act of harassment, intimidation or bullying.

    (2) A school employee, student or volunteer who witnesses or has reliable information that a student has been subjected to an act of harassment, intimidation or bullying is encouraged to report the act to the appropriate school official designated by the school district's policy.

    (3) A school employee who promptly reports an act of harassment, intimidation or bullying to the appropriate school official in compliance with the procedures set forth in the school district's policy is immune from a cause of action for damages arising from any failure to remedy the reported act.

Section 6. School districts are encouraged to form harassment, intimidation or bullying prevention task forces, programs, and other initiatives involving school employees, students, administrators, volunteers, parents, guardians, law enforcement and community representatives.

Section 7. Sections 1 to 7 of this 2001 Act may not be interpreted to prevent a victim of harassment, intimidation or bullying from seeking redress under any other available law, whether civil or criminal. Sections 1 to 7 of this 2001 Act do not create any statutory cause of action.

Note. The bill was enrolled in the 71st Oregon Legislative Assembly—2001 Regular Session. It was passed by the Oregon State House of Representatives on May 17, 2001, and by the Oregon State Senate on May 30, 2001.

bullying, anti-harassment, and anti-intimidation policy and the completion of a school-based needs assessment are considered important first steps and "best practice" in effectively addressing the problem in schools (Olweus, 1991; Snell et al., 2002; Walker, Ramsey, & Gresham, 2004). Form 5.1 at the end of the chapter is a sample checklist and survey that is useful for school staff that are just starting this process. The checklist and survey items are drawn from materials provided by the U.S. Department of Education/Office of Civil Rights, and the National Association of Attorneys General (1999) as well as the literature and research on bullying and harassment (Olweus, 1991, 1993, 1994; Snell et al., 2002; Smith & Sprague, 2001, 2003). The first five items contain checklist indicators that typify the critical features of a comprehensive anti-bullying and anti-harassment policy. Items 6–14 comprise a staff survey designed to assess the incidence, prevalence, and responses to bullying and harassment in the educational setting; these items can function as a basic needs assessment. School personnel addressing the issues outlined in the checklist and survey items will find, in all likelihood, that they are in compliance with most of the legal guidelines and requirements that commonly comprise state and local policy today. It is, however, important that educators be familiar with their individual responsibilities in relation to district, local, state, and federal laws as they change and evolve. In addition to staff assessments, it is highly recommended that student surveys be conducted at some point each year in order to assess the incidence and frequency of bullying and harassment in the school (Smith & Sprague, 2003; Olweus, 1993). This recommendation reflects the finding that although even the most overt bullying and harassment behaviors are seldom seen by adults, they *are* witnessed or experienced by students on a daily basis. To that end, it is suggested that survey items 6–14 of the checklist and survey in Form 5.1 be adapted as a basic student survey.

CONCLUSION

Although there is a great deal of current emphasis on bullying and harassment problems in schools, these problems have been a major issue in schools and communities for a very long time. Public concern is just beginning to catch up with reality. We, as teachers, administrators, school staff, parents, and community members, should recognize that the antisocial behavioral characteristics commonly associated with bullying and harassment are part of a widespread behavior pattern among today's youth. Research has shown that among boys identified as bullies as early as second grade, up to 60% were found guilty of a felony by age 24 (Olweus, 1991). This finding documents the observation of Patterson that youth who adopt this behavior pattern are high-rate victimizers of others—and they are also victimized by their own behavior (Patterson, personal communication, 1988).

Outcomes for both boys and girls engaging in bullying and harassment tend to be dismal and grim. Severely aggressive behavior rarely has been found to change over time (Patterson, Reid, & Dishion, 1992; Reid, Patterson, & Snyder, 2002). Males and females engaging in antisocial conduct are likely to continue the cycle of violence and abuse inherent in bullying and harassment by exposing their own children to the attitudes, beliefs, values, and actions that replicate this undesirable behavior across generations (Wahler & Dumas, 1986). Unless children who chronically bully and harass others are exposed to interventions early on and are supported by parents or caregivers, it becomes extremely difficult to turn around this behavior pattern.

A need remains for further research and development in the area of bullying and harassment prevention technologies to build upon the solid work that has already taken place (see Espelage & Swearer, 2003; Juvonen & Graham, 2001). Teachers, school staff, and parents have a high stake in (and a legal responsibility for) alleviating the effects of bullying and harassment in today's schools. The scope of the problem is staggering and continues to worsen. Our recent survey findings (unpublished) indicate that up to 96% of elementary students are witnessing multiple instances of violent and threatening behavior during the course of 1 school year. Some students report that rude, hurtful, violent, and/or threatening actions are witnessed by the majority of students in the average school on a daily basis. The harmful negative impact of this constant bombardment is very serious. Gaining access to effective, research-based interventions for these problems is critical for educational professionals as well as parents and community members.

FORM 5.1. BULLYING, HARASSMENT, AND INTIMIDATION: SCHOOL-BASED POLICY CHECKLIST AND SELF-ASSESSMENT SURVEY

Checklist: What Has Been Done to Prevent BHI in Your School?
Survey: Is BHI a Problem in Your Building?

Instructions: Read the numbered question, then read and check the questions with which you most agree. Leave the questions with which you disagree. Check *all* choices with which you agree in cases where the question instructions indicate it is appropriate. Otherwise, when multiple choices are not indicated, check only the *one* question with which you *most* agree.

1. Do you have a specific policy against bullying, harassment, and intimidation and a written code of conduct that publicizes it?

   Do you have such a policy? ____

   Does the policy address all forms of BHI: sexual, racial/ethnic, sexual orientation, and differently abled? ____

   Does the policy contain a definition, procedures, sanctions, and prescribed method for notifying people? ____

   Is there a procedure whereby new employees and students are informed of the policy? ____

   Are there references to BHI in the student, staff, and parent handbooks? ____

   Are there references to BHI in the school discipline code? ____

   Are supervisors of student extracurricular activities, school-associated events, and job-training work sites notified of the BHI policy? ____

   Are vendors and salespersons visiting the district apprised of the BHI policy? ____

2. Do you have a grievance procedure to handle complaints about harassment and to monitor its effectiveness? (This may or may not be the same as other grievance procedures.)

   Do you have a reporting procedure for BHI? ____

   Do you have a grievance procedure for BHI? ____

   Does the grievance procedure provide an opportunity for informal consultation and, when appropriate, informal resolution before moving into formal procedures? ____

   Does the grievance procedure provide for impartial investigation that includes fact finding, careful review, due process, and opportunity for appeal? ____

(continued)

Does the grievance procedure include an appropriate remedy based on the severity of offense and institutional corrective action when there is a finding of BHI? ____

Has information about these procedures been disseminated to parents, staff, and students? ____

3. Are you prepared to receive and respond to complaints?

Are most staff members trained to take reports of BHI? ____

Are there staff members of both genders available to take reports and follow through, and are they balanced by ethnicity, race, and linguistic group? ____

Do all students and staff know the name and location of at least two staff members who are available? ____

Are those wishing to file a complaint allowed to go to any staff member with whom they feel comfortable? ____

Have staff members and investigators received regular yearly training? ____

Do the staff members meet on a regular basis to engage in group problem solving and to identify their needs for further training and support? ____

Are the staff members given released time from their regular duties to attend to report follow-up, investigation management, and record-keeping tasks? ____

Do the staff have access to training and legal advice regarding the proper processing of complaints and potential legal liability? ____

Do administrators work cooperatively with staff members: that is, are interventions, sanctions, and remedies actually applied? ____

Does the administration and school board receive regular statistical reports by the school regarding the number and type of formal and informal complaints filed and their disposition? ____

4. Do you foster an atmosphere of prevention by sensitizing students and staff to the issue of BHI? Does the definition of BHI make it clear that sexual, racial/ ethnic, sexual orientation, and differently abled harassment are included?

Does the district mission statement reflect a commitment to the value of mutual respect for all people? ____

Has there been a training program for administrators, staff, and interested parents in the past 2 years? ____

Has there been a training program for district employees, including job-training supervisors, in the past 2 years? ____

Has there been a training program for students in the past 2 years? ____

Do staff members model the use of appropriate language and behavior at all times? ____

(continued)

Are pamphlets and/or posters advising students and employees about the nature of BHI, the appropriate responses to it, and its legal implications easily found around the school? ____

Has a schoolwide conference or "speakout" been held to sensitize the school community to the issues of BHI? ____

Is information about preventing BHI and what to do if they occur a routine part of the K–12 curricula? ____

Do staff members promptly intervene in situations where they observe BHI? ____

Is offensive graffiti that violates the BHI policy promptly removed? ____

Do student leaders take an active role in the effort to prevent BHI? ____

Have events where BHI typically occur, such as "flipup" days and pep rally cross-dressing skits, been eliminated? ____

Have past incidents of BHI been resolved fairly and appropriately? ____

Do students and staff members feel comfortable talking openly about BHI incidents, problematic areas, and attitudes? ____

5. Have you reached out to populations of students known to be particularly vulnerable to BHI?

Have support groups been established for students enrolled in vocational or academic classes that are nontraditional for their gender, race, or ethnicity? ____

Are students who drop vocational or academic classes that are nontraditional for their gender, race, or ethnicity routinely surveyed to establish the reason for dropping and to determine whether BHI played any role in their decision? ____

Are student placement work sites routinely visited and evaluated for freedom from BHI? ____

6. Do you know of instances of harassment that have happened in your building? Yes ____ No ____

If yes, what kind of harassment was it? (Check all that apply.)

Sexual ____   Differently abled ____
Racial/ethnic ____   Other ____
Sexual orientation ____

If yes, was the harassment between
Student(s)/student(s) ____
Student(s)/staff ____
Staff/staff ____

(continued)

FORM 5.1. *(page 4 of 6)*

How many instances have you been aware of in the past year?

One ____   Two to five ____   Six or more ____

7. Do you know of instances of bullying that have happened in your school?
   Yes ____   No ____

   If yes, what kind of bullying was it? (Check all that apply.)

   Violence ____
   Intimidation ____
   * Rumors/lies/slander ____
   Theft ____
   Social threats ____
   Threats of physical violence ____
   Destruction of property ____

   Social isolation ____
   Mean-spirited teasing ____
   Inappropriate sexual contact—
     verbal ____
   Inappropriate sexual contact—
     physical ____
   Other ____

   How many instances have you been aware of or witnessed in the past 30 days?
   One ____   Two to five ____   Six or more ____

   How many instances have been reported to you by students in the past 30 days?
   One ____   Two to five ____   Six or more ____

8. Do you know of students who have dropped a class or had their grades affected because of BHI?   Yes ____ No ____
   How many instances have you heard of in the past year?
   One ____   Two to five ____   Six or more ____

9. Do you know of students who have stayed at or gone home because of BHI?
   Yes ____   No ____
   How many instances have you heard of in the past year?
   One ____   Two to five ____   Six or more ____

10. In cases of BHI that you know about, what did the victim do? (Check all that apply.)

    Ignored it ____
    Complained to school authorities ____
    Told perpetrator to stop ____
    Told an adult staff member ____
    Went along with it ____
    Replied in kind ____
    Had a fight ____
    Ran away ____

    Went home from school ____
    Cried ____
    Told his/her parent(s)/guardian(s) ____
    Tried to work it out peacefully/
      appropriately ____
    Told his/her friends/peers
    ____ Other

(continued)

121

11. What happened in cases of BHI that you know were reported to school authorities? (Check all that apply.)

The charge was found to be true ____   Action was taken against
Nothing happened ____   harasser ____
The charge was found to be   Do not know what happened ____
  false ____   Action was taken against the
The charge is still being   victim ____
  processed ____   Other ____

12. What happens when BHI occurs at school *and* there is an adult there or nearby who can see or hear what is going on? (Check all that apply.)

The adult stops it ____   The principal/dean punishes everyone
The adult reports it to the principal   present ____
  or dean ____   The principal/dean reminds everyone
The principal/dean does nothing ____   how to behave ____
The principal/dean tells the students   The principal/dean helps those
  to take care of it themselves ____   involved to solve their problems and
The principal/dean is too busy to do   get along ____
  anything ____   Other ____
The principal/dean punishes the
  perpetrators ____

13. In cases of BHI that you know of, if the victim did nothing, why do you think he or she did nothing? (Check all that apply.)

Did not want to hurt the   Thought it would make him/her
  perpetrator ____   uncomfortable with the
Did not know what to do ____   perpetrator ____
Did not think it was necessary to   Thought it would make it happen even
  report ____   more or worse ____
Was too embarrassed ____   Thought it would make the other
Did not think anything would be   students think negatively about him
  done ____   or her ____
Was afraid the perpetrator would get   Other ____
  even ____

14. How widespread do you think BHI is in your school?

It goes on all the time ____   It happens to a fair number of
It goes on most the time ____   students ____
It goes on about half the time ____   It happens to most students ____
It goes on occasionally ____   It happens to all students ____
It goes on very seldom ____   It does not happen ____
It does not happen in our school ____
It only happens to a few
  students ____

(continued)

122

15. Please check the categories that best apply to you.

       Male ____   Female ____

       Your race/ethnicity _____

       Your role in school _____

6

Screening and Identifying Behaviorally At-Risk Students

Purposes, Approaches, Outcomes, and Cautions

The use of proactive and systematic screening procedures to identify diseases, deficits, and disorders of various types is a professional practice that has a long tradition in U.S. society. Hearing and vision deficits, multiple types of cancer, heart disease, and reading failure are but a few of the conditions that have been the targets of public health screening efforts. Sophisticated tests and screening systems have been developed and validated that are used to detect either the presence or absence of some conditions (e.g., cancer) and pathological levels of others (e.g., hearing and vision deficits). These screening methods are an integral component of ensuring the public health and well-being. In addition, they are a key ingredient in achieving secondary and tertiary prevention outcomes. As a general rule, screening initiatives of this type are viewed as highly cost effective and desirable.

However, this policy has been anything but the case in the area of school-related behavior disorders (Kaufman, 1999, 2003, 2004). Resistance to the early, systematic screening of all students in order to proactively identify those in need of supports, services, and interventions for their emotional and behavioral problems has been a difficult "sell" within the public school system. Disadvantages frequently cited by educational decision makers as justifying such resistance include (1) stigmatizing, singling out, and pejoratively labeling students as having emotional or behavioral problems; (2) the inadvisability of identifying students for whom no services currently exist; (3) screening and treatment costs; (4) systemic bias among referral and screening agents;

(5) intrusiveness of procedures; and (6) the undesirable possibility of identifying large numbers of students for whom special accommodations and protections under the Individuals with Disabilities Education Act (IDEA), as well as specialized placements and services would have to be provided. Unlimited costs and lawsuits—two potential consequences associated with this last disadvantage—have tended to harden such resistance among school leaders and administrators. Plausible counterarguments to each of these perceived disadvantages exist and have been cited often in the public debate about the advisability of adopting proactive screening systems for identifying and providing services to students with behavioral disorders (see Kauffman, 2003). This issue has been, and continues to be, controversial; it is a source of considerable tension between general education, special education, and related services personnel who work in public schools.

A direct consequence of this resistance has been a substantial underidentification and underreferral of behaviorally at-risk children and youth for further evaluation, diagnosis, eligibility determination, provision of appropriate supports and services, and access to needed mental health resources. In a very important study involving two cohorts of 4,136 5-year-old Head Start children across 30 participating sites, Redden and colleagues examined special education identification rates for Head Start children in relation to emotional disturbance and related disabilities (Redden et al., 1999). These students were followed up in third grade, when evaluation of each child as being at risk for emotional disturbance and/or related disabilities was conducted using clinical cutoff scores on teacher rating instruments and individual testing completed in the spring of third grade. The special education eligibility of these children was determined from school records. Results indicated that only 31.8% of children considered to be at risk, using clinical diagnostic criteria, were actually identified by schools, and fewer than 6% of children at risk for emotional disorders were actually identified in the school category of emotional disorders. These outcomes document the pervasive underreferral of behaviorally at-risk students by school personnel and represent a serious problem that seems to be growing worse, if anything. Experts in child mental health consistently estimate that up to one-fifth of the school-age student population is in need of systemic services and supports to address their problems. Very often, schools provide the only gateway to accessing such services (Burns & Hoagwood, 2002).

Other research shows that students, in general, are far more likely to be referred to school-based services for academic than behavioral problems (Lloyd, Kauffman, Landrum, & Roe, 1991). Lloyd et al. (1991), for example, found that behavioral referrals ranked seventh on the top 10 reasons for teacher referral of students to special school services in a study of referral patterns in two Virginia school districts. The first six referral reasons involved learning and sensory problems. In a replication of these findings, Del'Homme, Kasari, Forness, and Bagley (1996) reported that students with academic problems were more likely to be referred to special education than were students with behavioral problems. Redden et al. (1999) note that many students with emotional and behavioral problems are likely referred and certified for special education in eligibility categories other than emotional disturbance (e.g., learning disabilities, speech and language impairment). These findings and this observation further buttress the case that schools are generally biased against the proactive identification and treatment of students who have serious emotional and behavioral problems. To date, the universal screening of all students, using cost-effective procedures, is a practice that has not been broadly adopted by school districts, even though there is clear evidence that such screening identifies students who have very serious emotional and behavioral problems (Walker, Severson, & Feil, 1995).

There has been a recent shift, however, in the posture of school personnel in relation to one aspect of these well-documented resistances. This change has developed as a result of intense concern about students who may hold the potential for violent actions at some point. The plethora of school shootings between 1994 and 1998, during which 188 violent deaths occurred in and around U.S. schools, has prompted an intense search for profiling systems that will enable the identification of potentially violent offenders among current student populations. There has been no shortage of individuals who have offered screening systems and checklists of symptoms that purport to achieve this goal—and with accuracy and precision! In our frank assessment, nothing could be further from the truth—or even a realistic possibility.

There is broad agreement among experts that no currently validated set of behavioral attributes exists that will allow the pre-identification of potentially violent offenders or school shooters on a case-by-case basis (LeBlanc, 1998). It has not been established that such pre-identification can be accomplished accurately or beyond chance expectation. Although it is possible to identify groups of youth (i.e. chronic juvenile offenders, gang members) who will have a higher rate of violent offending, over time, than nonjuvenile offenders, the decision-making process collapses when we go to the next step: predicting, on an individual basis, which of these youth will commit violent acts in the future. The downside of investing in these efforts is very serious and holds the real possibility of falsely victimizing innocent youth who are judged to match a behavioral profile considered to be predictive of future violent acts. They should be avoided at all costs—especially if the goal for their use is to exclude students from the schooling process because they represent a potential threat to school safety and security. Students' lives can be ruined on a wholesale basis from the stigma and reputational damage that would result from the use of such practices—not to mention the violation of their civil and legal rights.

Three groups of troubled students, whose problems have varying degrees of relationship to school security, can be targeted within school settings. These are (1) behaviorally at-risk students who come from high-risk backgrounds and bring a host of negative, destructive attitudes, beliefs, and actions with them to the schooling process; (2) students who make threats of serious aggression and violence toward others but do not follow through with their stated intentions; and (3) those who may or may not make public threats but actually engage in conspiratorial planning of school tragedies and sometimes carry them out, with tragic consequences, as occurred at Columbine High

School in Colorado and Thurston High School in Oregon. In our view, the needs and indicated actions of students within each of these groups should be systematically addressed; ignoring them in the hope that they will resolve themselves is the last option that should be considered. This chapter describes screening approaches that can be used to enable or facilitate achievement of this goal.

Before describing recommended screening approaches for use by school personnel, however, it is important to frame the critical issues and to describe the landscape around early risk factors and the warning signs of potential violence. We believe access to this knowledge base is essential for every adult working in today's schools.

RISK FACTORS AND THE WARNING SIGNS OF POTENTIAL VIOLENCE

Risk Factors

Risk factors, in this context, are those conditions and environmental elements that propel a youth toward violent activity and that increase its actual likelihood. There are two types of risks: proximal and distal. *Proximal risks* are embedded within the family context, whereas *distal risks* emerge from community and societal forces (e.g., exposure to community and media violence). Proximal risks are generally considered to be more influential or powerful than distal risks. The U.S. Surgeon General's report on youth violence (Satcher, 2001) notes that these risks also differ by developmental stage. For example, the strongest risk factors associated with violence during childhood are involvement in serious, but not necessarily violent, criminal behavior, substance use, male gender, proneness toward engaging in physical aggression, low family socioeconomic status or poverty, and parents with antisocial personalities. However, during adolescence, the list changes and the influence of family is largely supplanted by peer influences. Risks for violence during this period include weak ties to conventional peers, ties to antisocial or delinquent peers, belonging to a gang, and involvement in criminal acts. Unfortunately, increasingly greater numbers of our youth are exposed to many of these risks in their family and community contexts. This exposure sets them up for school failure and affiliation with deviant peer groups that are likely to exacerbate their problems and lead to highly destructive outcomes in later adolescence; these outcomes often include delinquency and, occasionally, acting as a perpetrator and/or a victim of violence.

The American Psychological Association (1993), in its seminal report on youth violence, identified four accelerators of violence that seem to increase the likelihood of its eruption among groups of behaviorally at-risk youth: (1) easy access to weapons, particularly handguns, (2) early involvement with drugs and alcohol, (3) association and affiliation with antisocial groups, and (4) pervasive exposure to violence in the media. Youth who come from at-risk backgrounds and display these characteristics may have an elevated risk of displaying violent behavior during their school careers. Patterson and his colleagues (Patterson, Reid, & Dishion, 1992; Reid, Patterson, & Snyder, 2002) have identified another high-risk group: those youth commonly referred to as chronic offenders (defined as having three or more arrests by age 12). These researchers found that violent activity was much more likely among groups of at-risk youth who (1) began offending by age 10 or less, (2) whose first arrest was for a relatively serious offense, and (3) who had at least three arrests by age 12.

Although it is important for educators to be fully informed about the family, neighborhood/community, and societal influences associated with youth violence, there is very little that they can do to directly address or prevent these causal influences. Many children begin their school careers woefully unprepared for the normal demands of schooling; worse, they bring attitudes, beliefs, and values that support antisocial forms of behavior. Schools and teachers are vulnerable to the damage these children can inflict and often do not cope well with the challenges they present. This chapter is intended to empower teachers and school personnel generally to more effectively screen, identify, and intervene with this student population, so that their problems can begin to show a pattern of deescalation rather than escalation over their school careers.

Warning Signs

Following the school shooting tragedy at Thurston High School in Springfield, Oregon, in 1998, in which the shooter murdered his parents, killed two of his classmates, and seriously wounded over 20 others, President Clinton commissioned the development of an early warning guide for use by educators in their efforts to make schools safer and cope with potential violence. A 25-member panel of experts was assembled to develop this guide; we were members of this panel. Over a 4-month period, the panel developed a document, *Early Warning/Timely Response: A Guide to Safe Schools* (EW/TR), which was mailed to all 125,000 public and private schools in the United States by September of 1998. This document met an important need at the time and has proved to be influential in the nation's response to the crisis induced by the school shooting tragedies of the 1990s. It also stimulated development of a broad-based federal funding initiative, Safe Schools/Healthy Students, in which consortia of school districts and community agencies are required to collaborate in addressing school safety issues and problems. The Institute on Violence and Destructive Behavior, under the leadership of one of us (J.R.S.), has provided extensive evaluation and technical assistance services to a number of grantees in the Northwest under auspices of this funding program.

The *Early Warning/Timely Response* guide specifies the signs that, when viewed in context, may identify a troubled student and can be quite useful in generating appropriate services, supports, and/or outside referrals. The EW/TR document distinguishes between early warning signs and imminent warning signs and also provides a set of guiding principles to help ensure that these signs will not be misinterpreted or abused.

Early Warning Signs

Early warning signs function much like the proverbial canary in the coal mine, in that they point to signs of trouble within a youngster. However, their presence does not necessarily mean that he or she is therefore likely to commit a violent act. Nevertheless, early warning signs usually sound an alarm that the student needs assistance for inter- or intrapersonal problems with which he or she is having difficulty coping. The more signs a student manifests, the greater the trouble he or she may be experiencing. Warning signs that raise the concern of key personnel can be quite valuable as an initial step in providing much-needed assistance.

The following indicators were compiled by the panel as early warning signs:

- Social withdrawal
- Excessive feelings of isolation and loneliness
- Excessive feelings of rejection
- Being a victim of violence
- Feelings of being picked on and persecuted
- Low school interest and poor academic performance
- Expression of violence in writings and drawings
- Uncontrolled anger
- Patterns of impulsive and chronic hitting, intimidating, and bullying
- History of discipline problems
- Past history of violent and aggressive behavior
- Intolerance for differences and prejudicial attitudes
- Drug and alcohol use
- Affiliation with gangs
- Inappropriate access to, possession of, and use of firearms
- Serious threats of violence

Parents, teachers, school counselors, and sometimes peers are the most likely informants of these warning signs, because they are in the best position to observe a child's characteristic behavior over time and to note atypical patterns or occurrences. It should be emphasized that these indicators should not be used as a behavioral checklist but rather as general guides to determine whether a child should be evaluated for potential problems.

Imminent Warning Signs

In contrast to early warning signs, *imminent warning signs* indicate that a student may be on the verge of behaving in a manner that is potentially dangerous to self and/or others. These signs involve or imply a threatening situation and are characterized by hostility and uncontrolled anger. The panel's view was that imminent signs cannot be ignored and require an immediate response. Essentially, these signs mark a crisis that should be treated as an emergency. Imminent warning signs include the following:

- Serious physical fighting with peers or family members
- Severe, uncontrolled rage for seemingly minor reasons or provocations
- Detailed threats of lethal violence
- Severe destruction of property
- Possession and/or use of firearms and other weapons
- Other self-injurious behaviors or threats of suicide

In addition to these danger signs, the panel defined two situations that *always* require an immediate response involving school authorities, mental health experts, and/or law enforcement officers: (1) when the student has developed a detailed plan to harm or kill others—especially if the student has a history of making threats and behaving in a very aggressive manner; and (2) when the student brings a firearm to school and threatens to use it. Both of these situations call for application of threat assessment protocols to determine their level of danger, likelihood of being implemented, and appropriate intervention.

Similarly, Trump (2000) has distinguished between "less serious" and "very serious" behavioral indicators of violence and threats to school safety. There is substantial overlap between the EW/TR imminent signs and the "very serious" ones identified by Trump (2000):

- Suicidal thoughts or attempts and related self-injury and harm
- Attempting to cause the death of, or serious physical harm to, another person
- Intentional abuse of animals
- Setting fires
- Hallucinations or other delusions
- Specific plans, especially detailed ones, for committing violence

Trump (2000) correctly notes that these signs do not represent a diagnostic checklist or protocol but *do* indicate the need for involvement of mental health professionals experienced in working with troubled, violence-prone youth. Interestingly, the perpetrator of the Thurston High School tragedy in Springfield, Oregon, had a known history of abusing animals (drowning cats in pool chemicals), hearing voices, and suicidal ideation. After the tragedy, he was diagnosed as having paranoid schizophrenia.

It is critical that educators be aware of these early and imminent warning signs because recognizing any of them puts educators on alert regarding what to watch for among students, in general, and particularly among behaviorally at-risk students. Prevention and timely intervention cannot occur in the absence of this knowledge. However, this information is easily abused, and it is not difficult to make critical mistakes in applying it. The EW/TR guide lists five key principles that provide some degree of protection against these outcomes:

1. Do no harm.
2. Understand that violence and aggression occur within a context that needs to be understood.
3. Avoid stereotypes.
4. View warning signs within a developmental context.
5. Understand that children typically exhibit multiple rather than isolated warning signs.

APPROACHES TO THE SCREENING AND IDENTIFICATION OF AT-RISK STUDENTS

From the available information on current school practices, it appears that both systematic identification procedures and consistency of outcomes are lacking for behaviorally at-risk students who may pose a risk to themselves and/or others (see Sprague & Walker, 2000; Walker, Nishioka, Zeller, Severson, & Feil, 2000). As a result, these students are often identified far too late in their school careers—and at a point when interventions are not only less successful but also come at increasing cost. Furthermore, at-risk students whose needs are ignored may perceive the school environment as uncaring and feel alienated from it—a perception that many of the school shooters shared in common.

As noted earlier, today's students increasingly come from backgrounds where they are exposed to risk factors that set them up for serious school adjustment problems and put them on a path to destructive outcomes in adolescence and young adulthood. These risks often include poverty, drug and alcohol use by parents and caregivers, family dysfunction, child neglect and abuse, deteriorating neighborhoods and communities that are crime ridden and sometimes characterized by high levels of violence, a lack of family monitoring, supervision, and discipline, and overexposure to media violence. There is little that schools can do to either pre-assess for, or to prevent, the exposure of K–12 students to such family and community-based risks; however, they must deal with the behavioral manifestations of them, which often pose serious challenges for school personnel. There are risks, however, associated with the school setting itself; experiences of low academic achievement and school failure, mean-spirited teasing and bullying, alienation and discrimination, and association/affiliation with antisocial peers (see Satcher, 2001, for a detailed description of risk factors associated with antisocial behavior, delinquency, and violence). Schools can and should do something to address these particular risk factors, which have everything to do with determining whether schooling serves as an overall protective or dangerous experience.

We recommend that educators consider four key approaches to the early screening and identification of students who display emotional and behavioral difficulties. These approaches can enable educators to assist at-risk students whose behavior sometimes signals the presence of serious problems requiring educational, psychological, and/or psychiatric intervention. The following approaches are an essential component of the arsenal of safety strategies that all schools should have in place:

1. Using systematic interventions designed to achieve prevention goals and outcomes, and student responses to them, as a basis for identifying those students who are in need of assistance for their problems.
2. Proactively implementing universal screening procedures on a regular basis to identify those students who suffer from either externalizing or internalizing behavioral challenges.
3. Analyzing archival school records as a means of identifying and profiling behaviorally at-risk students.
4. Applying threat-assessment procedures, as developed by the FBI and U.S. Secret Service, to determine the degree of danger and credibility of situations in which students make threats toward others in the school setting.

These approaches are described below and their applications within the school setting illustrated. Expected outcomes and cautions associated with these approaches are also discussed.

Early identification, as used in this context, contains two implications of salience for professional practice: (1) It is very important to detect the development of adjustment problems as early as possible in their trajectories, so that they can be successfully interrupted and the associated problem(s) addressed and (2) Equally important, it is imperative that access to intervention occurs early in the lives and schooling of at-risk children and youth. Early intervention to achieve prevention goals is very difficult to accomplish without early screening and detection.

Although each identification approach described in the following material can be used in isolation, it is recommended that combinations of them be considered as appropriate and feasible within particular school settings. LeBlanc (1998) has argued persuasively that screening approaches and methods for use in identifying antisocial, potentially violent youth should involve multiple agents or informants (parents, teachers, peers), multiple settings (home, school, community), and multiple methods (informant ratings, direct observation, archival records) whenever possible. Adopting these practices will facilitate better decision making and fewer errors in the screening and identification process.

USING PREVENTION-BASED INTERVENTIONS AS A MEANS OF IDENTIFYING BEHAVIORALLY AT-RISK STUDENTS

The U.S. Public Health Service has developed a classification schema governing its major approaches to prevention that includes primary, secondary, and tertiary types.

Primary prevention refers to the avoidance of harm through the adoption of wellness and vaccination practices that prevent health-related problems from developing. *Secondary prevention* refers to the reversal of harm through use of more intensive treatment of individuals with conditions that show the early signs of pathology. *Tertiary prevention* describes efforts to reduce harm associated with the most serious forms of disease or pathology. Walker and his associates (Walker et al., 1996) have adapted this model of prevention to the schooling context for the purposes of (1) establishing positive school climates, (2) providing a means to address the needs and problems of all students, and (3) achieving greater coordination among levels and types of intervention designed to address overall prevention goals. This adaptation has proven to be very popular with educators for its utility in developing positive behavior support strategies for schools. In the Walker et al. (1996) adaptation, prevention is viewed as a goal or outcome of intervention rather than as a process. Figure 6.1 provides a schematic overview of this model adapted for schools.

As a rule, universal interventions are used to achieve primary prevention goals and outcomes (e.g., fluoridating a community's water supply to prevent dental car-

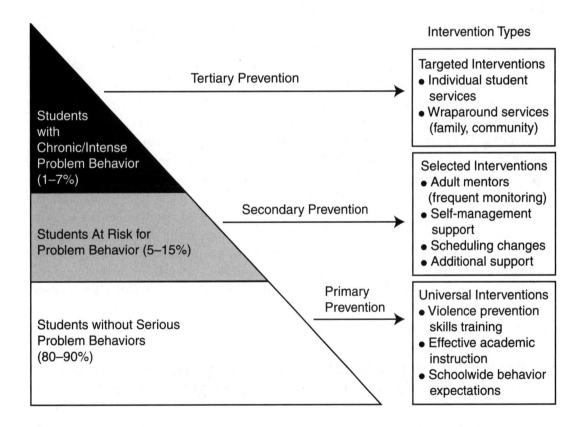

FIGURE 6.1. Schematic overview of types of school-based prevention.

ies). In the case of schools, primary prevention examples would include establishing schoolwide discipline programs (see Chapter 3), the universal teaching of violence prevention skills, bully-proofing the school, or implementing evidence-based instructional methods across all classrooms. Secondary prevention involves the provision of more intensive supports, services, and treatment to those students for whom the primary prevention strategy is insufficient. Interventions designed to achieve secondary prevention goals are usually referred to as *selected*, in that students select themselves out as requiring these extra supports and accommodations. At the secondary level, students are typically addressed on an individual basis or within small groups, where more intensive interventions can be applied. Finally, tertiary prevention efforts involve the most powerful interventions and supports available and typically require the resources and skills of professionals or agencies external to the school (e.g., mental health, child protection, social services). Interventions at this level are called *targeted*, and they are the most expensive of any included within this model.

This comprehensive prevention model makes it possible to address the needs of all students within any school: (1) those who are progressing normally, (2) those who show early signs of risk exposure, and (3) those who have severe and elevated levels of problem behavior. Furthermore, interventions designed to address these three student groupings can be coordinated so as to maximize their effectiveness and to optimize the use of available resources. Referring to Figure 6.1, the more students who can be maintained at primary and secondary levels of prevention, the better it is for all students and for the school's overall climate or culture.

Kellam and Rebok (1992) have argued for the use of universal prevention programs as the initial or first level of screening. That is, those students who are unresponsive to the primary prevention strategies and whose problems and needs persist are referred to secondary and/or targeted levels of prevention for treatment, as appropriate. This is an excellent and very fair method of screening, provided that the primary prevention strategies are appropriate, well matched to the problem or need, and implemented with acceptable fidelity. However, this method does require the careful monitoring of student response to the universal intervention and a willingness to provide assessments of those students for whom the intervention is insufficient. In our experience, screening of this type is more acceptable to school personnel because it avoids the objections associated with screening efforts implemented in the absence of intervention (e.g., stigmatization, lack of fairness, special treatment of certain students).

Students who have serious mental health needs and problems, or are bullied and teased frequently, or are highly aggressive in their peer interactions, or are oppositional/defiant in their relations with adults are likely to stand out within a school context that has a positive climate or culture, that is well managed and instructed, and that is regarded as orderly and inclusive of all students. These are among the students who should become the targets of secondary and tertiary prevention efforts.

UNIVERSAL SCREENING TO PROACTIVELY IDENTIFY STUDENTS WITH EXTERNALIZING AND INTERNALIZING BEHAVIOR PROBLEMS

As noted, teachers or parents and sometimes peers are usually the key informants to provide the first level of screening within universal screening systems geared toward the early detection of students experiencing problems of a behavioral, emotional, or social nature. Typically, their input is solicited in the form of a request to nominate and/or rate selected students from the pool of total students; for example, students may be asked to name peers who are teased or bullied, or teachers may be asked to name students who do not meet their academic or behavioral expectations. Occasionally, teachers are asked to rate all students within a classroom on selected dimensions, using a small number of items, as in the Drummond (1993) universal screening system for identifying students at risk for antisocial behavior. In the Drummond procedure, the teacher assigns a Likert rating, on a scale of 0–3, to indicate the frequency, for example, with which each student in the regular classroom "sneaks" or "lies." With this method, teachers can rate an entire classroom within a relatively short period of time. This intriguing matrix-rating procedure is described in greater detail in a later section.

In other instances, teachers are asked to identify problem students in their classes in relation to certain criteria (e.g., likelihood of school failure) and then to rate those students on a Likert rating scale of negative and/or positive behavioral attributes; the Social Skills Rating Scale by Gresham and Elliott (1990) is an example of one such instrument. Although there are potential problems with this approach, in that the teacher is both nominating and rating the same students, it is a very popular screening method used in schools (see Lane, 2003). Form 6.1 at the end of this chapter contains a nomination and rating procedure, developed by Hill M. Walker and his colleagues, for use by teachers in identifying students who have low school engagement.

Feil, Severson, and Walker (2002) recently contributed an extensive review of school-based screening practices, wherein they evaluated the roles and efficacy of teacher nominations and Likert ratings, critical behavioral events, *in vivo* behavioral observations, and archival school records. As part of this review, they described their work in the development, validation, and norming of a multiple gating approach to the screening and early detection of students who have school-related behavior disorders within the elementary age range. The following section discusses and reviews portions of this material.

Teachers' nomination, evaluation, and referral of at-risk students have been the subject of substantial controversy in the professional literature over the past two decades (Gerber & Semmel, 1984; Gresham, Lane, MacMillan, & Bocian, 1999; Walker, Severson, & Feil, 1995). Feil et al. (2002) noted that some authors argue that a teacher's referral behavior is driven primarily by the desire to be rid of troublesome, difficult-to-teach students toward the goal of creating more easily managed, homogeneous classrooms. A counterargument is that teachers are motivated by their good-faith interest in securing assistance for students whose problems and needs exceed their perceived skill levels and accommodation capacities (see Gerber & Semmel, 1984). We believe teacher referral practices are governed more by the latter consideration than the former. Nevertheless, there are a number of potential problems associated with an exclusive reliance on teacher nomination and referral of students for specialized services; for example, differences in behavioral tolerances among teachers, underreferral that leads to lack of service, and insensitivity to internalizing problems. In our view, these problems should be regarded as potential risks and cautionary points in the screening/identification process.

Teacher Nominations

If teacher nominations are the only school-based approach used to meet the needs of students with behavior problems, then the idiosyncratic behavioral standards, tolerance levels, and judgmental biases of referring teachers are free to operate in an unconstrained fashion across classrooms and school settings. Long-established empirical evidence indicates that regular teachers vary tremendously on these dimensions (Brophy, 1986; Brophy & Evertson, 1981; Gerber & Semmel, 1984; Walker, 1986). Thus, students with identical behavioral characteristics and needs may have very different probabilities of referral by individual teachers due to this teacher variability. The underidentification and referral of behaviorally at-risk students continues to plague school-based prevention/intervention efforts and is a critical problem; yet school administrators go to what appear to be extraordinary lengths to prevent the overreferral of students with serious behavior disorders (see Feil et al., 2002; Kauffman, 2003, 2004).

Teacher Ratings

Teacher ratings of student behavior, based on Likert scales, have been a popular, albeit unsystematic, approach in the evaluation of students referred for social, emotional, and behavioral problems (see Merrell, 2001, 2003). Such Likert scales typically ask the rater to assess students' behavior along three-, five-, or seven-point dimensions of problem frequency or severity. Hundreds of such scales are in use, and evaluations of many of them can be accessed through the *Fifteenth Mental Measurements Yearbook* (Plake, Impara, & Spies, 2003), which annually reviews newly developed scales. In addition to their unsystematic use, critics of teacher rating instruments point to their global and relatively crude assessment properties (e.g., "How many fidgets are there in a rating of *pretty much*"?). Others argue that the sensitivity of teacher ratings pale in comparison to more direct measures, such as *in vivo* behavioral observations.

In spite of these criticisms, teacher ratings continue to be a widely used and important source of information in child screening, identification, and evaluation processes. When used in combination with other assessment measures, they are especially valuable tools and can yield useful information that has utility for both screening/identification and outcome assessment purposes. These ratings have the advantage of defining and pinpointing the behavioral content of a student's perceived adjustment problems. In addition, the ratings can be standardized to enable valid social comparisons referenced to normative age and gender scores. Merrell (2001) has pointed out that Likert behavioral ratings have a number of additional advantages. They (1) are relatively inexpensive; (2) provide essential information on low-frequency behavioral events of potential importance; (3) are relatively objective and reliable, especially when compared to interview and projective assessment methods; (4) can assess individuals who are unable to contribute self-reports; (5) take into account the many observations and judgments of child behavior made by social agents within natural settings over the long term; and (6) reflect the judgments of expert social informants who are familiar with the student's behavioral characteristics (i.e., parents, teachers, peers).

Case Example of a Cost-Efficient Screening Approach Using Teacher Ratings

Drummond (1993) has developed an intriguing matrix system, based on Likert teacher ratings, to screen entire classrooms of students for their risk status in relation to antisocial behavior patterns. Drummond's Student Risk Screening Scale (SRSS) is a cost-efficient procedure for quickly screening whole classrooms. A matrix format is used; it has seven behavioral descriptors across the top of the rating form and students' names down the left side. The classroom teacher assigns every student a Likert rating, ranging from 0 = never to 3 = frequently, for each of these seven items: (1) stealing; (2) lying, cheating, sneaking; (3) behavior problems; (4) peer rejection; (5) low academic achievement; (6) negative attitude; and (7) aggressive behavior. Teachers compare each student against all others in the classroom as they rate each item. That is, *all* students are rated on item 1, then 2, and so forth. The SRSS is brief, research based, easily understood, valid, and cost efficient.

The major advantages of the SRSS are that (1) all students are systematically screened and evaluated and (2) normative social comparisons are facilitated by requiring the teacher to evaluate all students on each item at the same time, rather than rating individual students on a series of items on a case-by-case basis. The SRSS thus affords every student an equal chance to be evaluated in relation to each of the seven SRSS items simultaneously. A matrix system of this type is also ideally suited for the classwide assessment and pre–post evaluation of whole-class instruction on a series of social skills. A more complete description of the SRSS and its potential applications is provided in Walker, Colvin, and Ramsey (1995) and Walker, Ramsey, and Gresham (2004).

Teacher Ratings of Social Skills

Teacher Likert ratings of key social skills that assess critical dimensions of school and classroom adjustment have been widely used as initial screening and program evaluation measures within school settings during the past two decades (Merrell, 2003). Three of the more popular and technically adequate social skills measures designed for this purpose are (1) the Social Skills Rating Scale (SSRS; Gresham & Elliott, 1990), (2) the School Social Behavior Scales (SSBS; Merrell, 1993, 2002b), and (3) the Scales of Social Competence and School Adjustment (SSCSA; Walker & McConnell, 1995a). Brief descriptions of the rating formats, psychometric characteristics, and item content follow.

THE SOCIAL SKILLS RATING SCALE

The SSRS is a multicomponent social skills assessment system that is based on social–ecological principles. The SSRS is the only social skills rating system that obtains information from three key informant sources: teachers, parents, and the self-reports of students. This multi-informant and multiple-setting feature is one of the greatest strengths of the SSRS.

The SSRS spans the age-developmental range from preschool through grade 12 and is divided into three scales: preschool (ages 3–5), elementary (grades K–6), and secondary (grades 7–12). Each item is rated on a 3-point frequency scale (0 = never, 1 = sometimes, 2 = very often) according to the rater's estimate of how often the behavior described in the item occurs. In addition, classroom teachers are asked to rate the social importance of each item, according to how critical or important it is to a successful classroom adjustment. The SSRS contains five, factorially derived social skills domains; these form the basis for its subscales. These domains are: *cooperation, assertion, responsibility, empathy,* and *self-control.* Three of these domains (cooperation, assertion, and self-control) are replicated across student, teacher, and parent instrument forms. The SSRS also contains three subscales that measure problem behavior (externalizing, internalizing, and hyperactivity).

The SSRS was initially standardized on over 4,000 students enrolled in grades K–12 settings. The standardization sample was stratified by race and ethnicity and appears to be representative of the student demographic characteristics that typify today's schools. The SSRS has excellent psychometric characteristics and technically adequate estimates of its reliability and validity, as reported in the SSRS technical manual. The SSRS has become the gold standard for social skills assessments in school and home contexts and has been extensively researched by other investigators. It is a highly recommended instrument.

THE SCHOOL SOCIAL BEHAVIOR SCALES

The SSBS is a 65-item rating scale for teachers that provides measures of two "broadband" constructs: *social competence* and *antisocial behavior*. The scale covers the K–12 age-developmental range and is divided into two forms. Form A has 32 items and assesses social competence via three subscales: interpersonal skills, self-management skills, and academic skills. Form B assesses antisocial behavioral dimensions via 33 items and three subscales: hostile–irritable, antisocial–aggressive, and demanding–disruptive. Each item on Forms A and B is rated by the teacher on a 5-point Likert scale that is frequency based (i.e., 1 = never to 5 = frequently). The two scales were standardized on a national sample of 1,855 students in grades K–12.

The psychometric properties of the SSBS are excellent. Internal consistency estimates are typically above .90 and test–retest reliability estimates over a 3-week period range from .76 to .83 for the social competence scale and from .60 to .73 for the antisocial scale. Extensive studies of the convergent and discriminant validity of the SSBS have been conducted and are reported in the technical manual.

Merrell (2002a) has also developed a preschool version of the SSBS, known as the Preschool and Kindergarten Behavior Scale (PKBS). This scale was designed for completion by preschool teachers, caregivers, and other providers who are in a position to judge the social behavior of preschool-age children. The PKBS is a 76-item scale designed to measure social skills and problem behavior; items are rated on a 4-point Likert frequency-based scale. It was normed on over 2,000 preschoolers. Extensive information on the technical adequacy of the PKBS is contained in the scale's manual.

The SSBS and PKBS are highly recommended for screening, identification, and program evaluation purposes in the areas of social effectiveness and problem behavior. These scales provide comprehensive coverage of the social–behavioral adjustment domains that are so critical to school success.

THE SCALES OF SOCIAL COMPETENCE AND SCHOOL ADJUSTMENT

The SSCSA was designed for exclusive use by classroom teachers to assess the social skills of students in grades K–12 (Walker & McConnell, 1995a). The scales focus on positively stated social skills that support teacher- and peer-related forms of school adjustment; no subscales assessing antisocial or problem behavior are included. An elementary school version of the SSCSA (K–6) consists of 43 items and three subscales (teacher-preferred social behavior, peer-preferred social behavior, and school adjustment). The adolescent scale version (grades 7–12) has 53 items and four subscales, including the same three from the elementary version plus an empathy subscale. A 5-point Likert frequency-based scale is used to rate the items (1 = never occurs to 5 = frequently occurs). The SSCSA was normed on a national sample of approximately 2,000 cases.

Extensive studies of the SSCSA have been conducted on its validity and reliability. Seven types of validity have been investigated for the scales. Internal consistency estimates are typically in the low to mid .90s, and test–retest reliability over a 3-week period ranges from the low .80s to the low .90s. The SSCSA appear to be relatively sensitive to intervention and treatment effects (see Walker & McConnell, 1995a).

The California Department of Mental Health has used this scale extensively in evaluating its Early Mental Health Initiative for behaviorally at-risk children who are just beginning their school careers. The SSCSA elementary scale version has been the primary tool used for conducting this evaluation process over the past 7 years. A database that contains over several hundred thousand cases currently exists on the scale, as used within California schools.

The SSCSA scale is considered to have robust psychometric properties. It has been a frequently used instrument in studies that investigate and evaluate problem behavior within the schooling context.

Behavioral Observations

Behavioral observations recorded in natural settings (e.g., homes, classrooms, playgrounds, hallways) remain the preferred method of most related services professionals for assessing the behavior problems of students. In typical school usage, the teacher referral process requires that a school psychologist, or other related services professionals, directly observe the target student in a setting or context in which the problem behavior occurs (i.e., the referral setting). The main purpose of this observation is to confirm or disconfirm the accuracy and validity of the teacher referral. A wide range of coding systems and recording procedures are used to accomplish this observation. However, the vast majority of observational instruments do not have adequate technical data or information to support their use. In addition, most of these codes lack local, state, or national norms that are needed to make social comparisons among students.

Naturalistic behavioral observations are also vulnerable to the observer bias and expectancy effects that can be induced by the observer's prior knowledge of the case. Furthermore, direct observations are time consuming and labor intensive, in that they usually require considerable planning and careful monitoring to be conducted effectively (see Merrell, 2001).

In spite of these downsides, naturalistic behavioral observations remain popular among school professionals. These observations do have an important role to play in the screening/identification process if they are incorporated into a comprehensive assessment process that involves less-expensive measures (e.g., teacher nominations, rankings, ratings, archival records searches). We do not recommend the use of observation in isolation but rather as an important part of a multiagent, multimethod, and multiplesetting assessment approach (Merrell, 2003). A model screening-identification procedure incorporating these features and designed for use with students experiencing school-related behavior disorders is described in the next section.

Since 1985, Walker and his colleagues have been operating a systematic program of research focused on the goal of developing, validating, and norming a proactive, universal screening system for elementary-age (grades K–6) students who are experiencing school-related behavior disorders. The Systematic Screening for Behavior Disorders (SSBD) procedure was developed and field tested to accomplish this goal (see Walker & Severson, 1990). Walker and Severson (1990) developed the SSBD screening procedure based on a conceptual model and corresponding empirical findings indicating that children's problem behavioral characteristics can be divided reliably into *externalizing* (e.g., aggressive, hyperactive, noncompliant, antisocial) and *internalizing* (e.g., shy, phobic, depressed, anxious, isolated from peers) dimensions (see Achenbach, 1991; Ross, 1980). The SSBD was patterned after screening models developed and validated by Greenwood, Walker, Todd, and Hops (1979) for the preschool screening of children at risk for social withdrawal, and by Loeber, Dishion, and Patterson (1984) for the screening of adolescents at risk for later delinquency. The SSBD is a proactive, universal screening procedure that gives each student an equal chance to be screened and identified for either externalizing or internalizing behavior disorders. The SSBD procedure consists of three screening stages or "gates," where movement through each gate is required for consideration at the next stage. Most students are screened out at the first gate because they do not meet the behavioral criteria necessary to proceed to the next phase of screening. Walker and Severson began their first trial testing of the SSBD in the mid-1980s and conducted extensive research (supported by a series of federal grants) on this screening system prior to its publication in 1990 (Walker & Severson, 1990).

Figure 6.2 illustrates the three screening stages of the SSBD. At gate 1, teachers are asked to think about all students in their class and to nominate those students whose characteristic behavior patterns most closely match either the externalizing or internalizing behavioral definitions provided for them. The three highest-ranked externalizing students and the three highest-ranked internalizers then move to screening stage (i.e., gate) 2, where their behavior is more specifically rated by the teacher on a 33-item Critical Events Index (CEI) and on both an adaptive (11 items) and a maladaptive (12 items) Likert rating scale (Combined Frequency Index; CFI) that requires estimates of frequency of occurrence.

Students who exceed national normative cutoff scores on these measures proceed to gate 3, where they are observed in classroom and playground settings. Using a direct observation procedure, a school professional (school psychologist, counselor, or behavioral specialist) observes and codes each target child's behavior for two 20-minute sessions in the regular classroom. A stopwatch measure of academic engaged time (AET) is used for the classroom observations. A 10-second partial-interval code (peer social behavior; PSB) that records the level, quality, and distribution of the target student's peer-related social behavior at recess, is used to

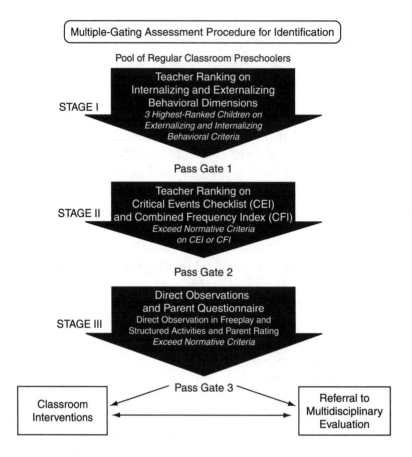

FIGURE 6.2. SSBD multiple-gating procedure. Adapted from Feil, Severson, and Walker (1994). Adapted by permission of the authors.

assess the student's playground behavior during the two 20-minute sessions. Normative data for the stage-2 instruments consist of over 4,000 cases representing the U.S. census zones. The SSBD user's manual also provides normative observation data for the AET and PSB codes involving over 1,300 cases—also collected across the U.S. census zones.

Those students who exceed national normative cutoff points on the AET and PSB codes are considered to have serious problems and are referred for further evaluation to specialized, school-based services. As a rule, an archival records search is conducted at this point to provide confirmation of the results of the screening/ identification process and to serve as another source of information for decision making.

The first two screening stages of the SSBD can be completed by the classroom teacher in approximately 1 hour. This screening procedure typically identifies one externalizer in every classroom and one internalizer in every two or three classrooms. The time involved in conducting SSBD screening assessments increases as one moves through the stages; however, the number of students who are the targets of those assessments is greatly reduced from stages 1 to 3. It is recommended that universal SSBD screenings be conducted twice a year (e.g., in October and February) to identify students in need of intervention supports and services, to maximize the sensitivity of school staff to initial behavior problems in the fall, and to detect emerging behavior problems later in the school year. The SSBD has been extensively researched and has excellent psychometric properties (see Walker & Severson, 1990).

ANALYZING ARCHIVAL SCHOOL RECORDS

If the early preschool detection of behavior problems is not possible, school records can provide an additional valuable source of screening information. Archival school records that accumulate as a natural part of the schooling process provide a rich and inexpensive information source regarding a range of school adjustment problems—as well as a record of the manner in which the schools tried to cope with such problems. Because these records accrue as an ordinary part of the schooling process, they are relatively unobtrusive and far less reactive than typically recorded assessments (e.g., teacher ratings, *in vivo* behavioral observations, sociometric measures).

Walker and his colleagues have developed the School Archival Records Search (SARS) procedure (see Walker, Block-Pedego, Todis, & Severson, 1991) to accomplish the coding, analysis, and aggregation of archival school records. SARS provides for the systematic coding of 11 variables, which can then be analyzed individually or aggregated into domain scores that provide profiles of student status in three areas of school adjustment: *disruption, needs assistance,* and *low achievement.* The individual SARS variables that are coded include the following: *number of different schools attended, days absent, low achievement, grades retained, academic/behavioral referrals, current Individualized Educational Program (IEP), nonregular classroom placement, Title I designation, referrals out of school, negative narrative comments,* and *school discipline referrals.* In the context of schooling, archival school records are the closest proxy we have for the police contacts and juvenile records that are used in evaluating delinquency prevention programs and in validating measures that purport to predict later delinquent acts. Analyzing archival school records is, in a sense, a form of educational archeology in that artifacts of past actions are used to reach important conclusions about the school, its students, and the school's efforts to cope with problems experienced by the student population.

Disciplinary referrals to the front office of students who are involved in behavioral episodes, as reflected in archival school records, have emerged as a very useful measure for assessing overall school status and for identifying student groups and individuals who are in need of behavioral supports and intervention (see Sugai, Sprague, Horner, & Walker, 2000; Walker, Stieber, Ramsey, & O'Neill, 1990). Sugai et al. have conducted extensive research on this topic during the past 5 years. Most recently, Sugai et al. (2000) reported normative data profiles on disciplinary referrals involving a sample of 11 elementary schools and 9 middle/junior high schools. These elementary schools averaged 0.5 disciplinary referrals per student per school year. At the middle/junior high school level, this level of disciplinary referrals was a very common occurrence. In the Sugai et al. study, the elementary schools averaged 566 students enrolled and 283 disciplinary referrals within a school year; the middle/junior high schools averaged 635 students and 1,535 disciplinary referrals within a school year.

These authors also analyzed some of the patterns that existed within this pool of disciplinary referrals. Based on this analysis, they argue that these patterns can guide the direction and focus of intervention approaches for addressing chronic behavior problems within the school setting (i.e., targeting the whole school, small groups, and/or individual students). For example, at the elementary level, Sugai et al. (2000) found that the top 5% of students with the most discipline referrals also accounted for 59% of total disciplinary referrals within the school; at the middle/junior high level, the top 5% accounted for 40% of all discipline referrals. These figures closely parallel outcomes for juvenile crime, where 6–8% of juveniles typically account for 60–65% of all delinquent acts (Loeber & Farrington, 1998b). According to Sugai et al., elementary-age students with five or more disciplinary referrals within a school year are considered to be behaviorally at risk; those with 10 or more such referrals are considered to be chronic discipline problems and possibly severely at risk for both in-school and out-of-school destructive outcomes.

Recording and utilizing disciplinary referrals to identify at-risk students and to guide intervention applications requires the computerization of school records. Horner and his associates have developed the School-Wide Information System (SWIS) procedure, which is a web-based computer application for entering, organizing, and reporting office discipline referrals found within school records (May et al., 2001). The SWIS computerization of discipline referrals is a valuable tool for use by teachers and school administrators in collecting and analyzing discipline-related information. One of the advantages of the SWIS procedure is that it systematizes and standardizes the process of documenting, recording, and reporting disciplinary referrals.

Form 6.2 at the end of the chapter is the SWIS Office Referral Form, which is completed for each disciplinary referral made by a teacher to the school office. The SWIS referral form notes the location, specific problem behavior, possible motivation(s) for the behavior, the resulting administrative decision, and other persons who were involved in the incident. Parents are asked to sign and date the referral form to indicate that they have knowledge of the incident, the referral, and its disposition.

SWIS is an important advance in the computerization of archival school records in that it allows individual schools to develop their own profile in relation to disciplinary practices and their resulting effects. It also can be used as a measure of certain aspects of school reform efforts, as a measure of the school's climate, as a pre–post measure of schoolwide interventions, and as a vehicle for guiding and targeting allocation of intervention resources to small groups and individuals. It is recommended as a schoolwide behavioral screening device with which to identify those students who are experiencing serious to chronic school adjustment problems.

APPLYING THREAT ASSESSMENT PROCEDURES WITHIN SCHOOL SETTINGS

Threat assessment refers to an investigative and evaluative process that is applied when an individual makes an apparently credible threat to commit a violent act against others (Walker, et al., 2004). The FBI and the U.S. Secret Service both have long histories and vast experience with evaluating/analyzing threats and have each developed processes for dealing with them. The FBI and the Secret Service have applied their threat assessment procedures to 18 and 37 school shooting incidents, respectively. These two agencies have provided detailed accounts of their procedures and guidelines in two highly recommended documents (see *The School Shooter: A Threat Assessment Perspective* [O'Toole, 2000] and *Threat Assessment in Schools: A Guide to Managing Threatening Situations and Creating Safe School Climates* [Fein et al., 2002]).

Though the FBI and Secret Service approaches share many common features, they differ in important ways. The FBI codes threats into four categories: *direct, indirect, veiled,* and *conditional*; these are rated low, medium, or high in terms of their likelihood. Threats that appear plausible and that present many specific details as to time and place are considered most likely to occur. Such threats prompt application of the FBI threat assessment process, which consists of assessing the following components: (1) the personality of the student, (2) family dynamics, (3) school dynamics and the student's role in them, and (4) social dynamics. Information gathered in each of these domains is analyzed in reaching a conclusion about the threat's credibility and making decisions about appropriate actions to instigate in order to cope with the threat.

The Secret Service distinguishes between a student who *makes* a threat and a student who *poses* a threat. This agency conducted extensive analyses of 37 school shootings and reported its findings in a widely disseminated document. These findings were used as a basis for identifying five principles that provide a foundation for the threat assessment process:

1. Targeted violence is the final step in an understandable process of thinking and acting.
2. Targeted violence involves an interaction between the perpetrator, the situation, the setting, and the target.
3. A skeptical and investigative mind-set is critically important to the threat assessment process.

4. Successful threat assessment rests upon documentable facts rather than traits or assumed characteristics.
5. A systems approach should guide threat assessment processes.

Some of the key findings compiled by the Secret Service investigative process include:

1. Targeted violence in school settings rarely involves sudden, impulsive acts.
2. There is no accurate or useful "profile" of students who engage in targeted school violence.
3. Many attackers reported being bullied, persecuted, or aggrieved by others, especially peers, prior to their attack.
4. Others nearly always know about an attack beforehand.
5. Most attacks have been prevented by other than law enforcement actions or intervention.

Recently, the Virginia Youth Violence Project at the University of Virginia released a threat assessment profile that shows great promise (see Cornell & Sheras, 2003). The protocol contains a set of specific guidelines for schools to follow in conducting threat assessments; these guidelines were field tested over a 2-year period. A key feature of this approach is that it allows school administrators to readily identify the small proportion of cases (fewer than 10%, as a rule) that require an extensive response. The protocol has been tested on 188 cases involving school-based threats over a 3-year field test. Information about this protocol can be accessed at *youthviolence.edschool.virginia.edu*.

In our view, all school officials and law enforcement personnel concerned with school safety should be thoroughly familiar with the content of the FBI and Secret Service approaches to threat assessment. Threats provide a red-flag opportunity to prevent potentially tragic acts. Many threats do not pose a serious danger to the school setting. Distinguishing real from frivolous threats remains a significant challenge and a heavy responsibility of school personnel.

CONCLUSION

The concept of proactive and universal screening/identification has a powerful history in the prevention of undesirable outcomes in a range of fields—most notably, medicine. In our view, schools substantially underutilize the technology that has developed over the past several decades in the area of behavioral screening and early detection of school adjustment problems. To a very large extent, effective prevention initiatives and efforts are hamstrung when the benefits and efficacy of proactive and universal screening are ignored.

We have recommended four major approaches to effective screening and identification of students experiencing school-based problems. Each approach has advantages and disadvantages; however, we believe the advantages of each method recommended far outweigh its associated disadvantages or costs. Two of these approaches (intervention-based screening and multiple gating, universal screening) are geared toward the proactive early detection of problems; they seek to provide each student with an equal opportunity to be identified for significant problems—an outcome that does not occur all that often, given current school practices. The other two approaches (analysis of archival school records and application of threat assessment procedures) are reactive in nature and occur after the fact. However, they both make it possible to respond to chronic and/or potentially dangerous situations posed by certain students. Ideally, all of these approaches should be considered for integration and coordination within a full-service school dedicated to serving the needs of all its students.

FORM 6.1. ASSESSING SCHOOL ENGAGEMENT AND WALKER–SEVERSON SCHOOL ENGAGEMENT INDEX

Hill M. Walker and Herbert H. Severson
Institute on Violence and Destructive Behavior
University of Oregon

The purpose of the following risk index is to:

1. Identify students early in their school careers who appear to be weakly engaged in the process of schooling using teacher judgement as an initial screening measure.

2. Systematically evaluate the social, behavioral, and academic status of such students using standardized, archival school records–search procedures.

3. Collect additional information that may influence the ultimate probability of school dropout (parental SES levels, social resiliency, the availability of social support networks, etc.).

The authors believe that the variable of *school engagement* is a powerful predictor of later school dropout and that dropout represents the ultimate expression of lack of school engagement. Further, students can be ordered very accurately on this dimension by their regular teachers in the elementary grades and possibly as early as grade one. This capability makes it possible to identify very early in their school careers those students who appear to be at risk for *low school engagement, school adjustment and academic failure*, and ultimately, *school dropout*. It is likely that many early school-leavers follow this path in a sequential, predictable fashion. The earliest possible identification of such students would make it feasible to interrupt this escalating chain or path of failure and to intervene effectively with it.

Rater Instructions

Step One. Please read the following definition of *school engagement*, which contains examples of both high and low engagement with the schooling process. A careful understanding of this definition is essential to your accurate identification of potential at-risk students.

Definition of School Engagement

The degree to which students are *actively engaged in the schooling process* varies substantially among current school populations. The more actively the student is engaged, the more likely she/he is to be successful in school. Actively engaged students are more likely to be characterized by *high achievement, timely completion of assigned tasks, a sense of independence and personal responsibility, a strong commitment to the value of schooling, positive interactions with peers and adults, a*

(continued)

capacity for being well-organized, and high levels of self-esteem and confidence. In contrast, a profile of the student with *low* school engagement would be characterized by the following behavioral attributes: *poor social skills, alienation from or hostility toward school, a nonexistent or weak social-support system, academic failure, lack of involvement in and commitment to the daily routines of schooling, ignoring and/or noncompliance with adult-imposed school rules, and a general failure to conform to adult expectations for behavior and achievement.*

Step Two. Using the behavioral profile of school engagement you just read, select the 5–10 students from your class whom you think are the *least engaged* in school. Rate each student on the behavioral characteristics listed in the left margin of the attached rating form. Please rate the student(s) on *each* behavioral characteristic listed.

Please use the following rating dimension in your appraisal of student status on each of the attributes listed:

1 = The behavior is *not* characteristic or true of the student.
3 = The behavior is *moderately* characteristic or true of the student.
5 = The behavior is *very* characteristic or true of the student.

Example:	Not descriptive or true	Moderately descriptive or true		Very descriptive or true	
1. Student rarely participates in group free-time activities with peers.	1	2	3	④	5

WALKER–SEVERSON SCHOOL ENGAGEMENT INDEX

Teacher _____ School _____ Grade ____ Date _____
Student Name _____

Rate each behavioral attribute listed by circling the number that best reflects your judgment.

	Not true		Moderately true		Very true
1. Student fails to complete classroom assignments.	1	2	3	4	5
2. Student attendance is erratic.	1	2	3	4	5

(continued)

	Not true		Moderately true		Very true
3. Student is socially rejected by peers.	1	2	3	4	5
4. Student breaks school rules.	1	2	3	4	5
5. Student lacks enthusiasm about school.	1	2	3	4	5
6. Student avoids extracurricular activities at school.	1	2	3	4	5
7. Student seems to have a negative attitude toward school.	1	2	3	4	5
8. Student displays sad affect and appears unhappy much of the time.	1	2	3	4	5
9. Student has no or few friends.	1	2	3	4	5
10. Student has issues outside school that interfere with school performance (frequent moves, homelessness, poverty, family problems).	1	2	3	4	5
11. Student displays bizarre or unusual forms of behavior.	1	2	3	4	5
12. Student shows evidence of alcohol, tobacco, or other illegal substance experimentation and use.	1	2	3	4	5
13. Student appears to have low self-esteem.	1	2	3	4	5
14. Student tends to affiliate with other students who also have low levels of school engagement.	1	2	3	4	5
15. Student is poorly motivated to achieve academically.	1	2	3	4	5

Total Score _____

FORM 6.2. OFFICE REFERRAL FORM

Name: _____

Date: _____ **Time:** _____

Teacher: _____

Grade: K 1 2 3 4 5 6 7 8

Referring Staff: _____

Location:

Playground	Library
Cafeteria	Bathroom
Hallway	Arrival/Dismissal
Classroom	Other _____

Problem Behavior	Possible Motivation	Administrative Decision

Minor
  Inappropriate language
  Physical contact
  Defiance
  Disruption
  Property misuse
  Other _____
Major
  Abusive language
  Fighting/physical
    aggression
  Over defiance
  Harassment/tease/taunt
Other _____
	Obtain peer attention
	Obtain adult attention
	Obtain items/activities
	Avoid peer(s)
	Avoid adult
	Avoid task or activity
	Don't know
	Other _____
		Loss of privilege
		Time in office
		Conference with student
		Parent contact
		Individualized instruction
		In-school suspension
		  (___ hours/days)
		Out of school suspension
		  (___ hours/days)
		Other _____

Others involved in incident:

None	Substitute
Peers	Unknown
Staff	Other
Teacher	

If peers were involved, list them _____

Other comments:

_____

_____

I need to talk to the student's teacher ____

I need to talk to the administrator ____

Parent Signature: _____ **Date:** _____

All minors are filed with classroom teacher. Three minors equal a major.

_____

From May et al. (2001). Reprinted by permission of the authors.

7

Supporting Antisocial
and Potentially Violent Youth

with VICKI NISHIOKA

Implementation of effective and evidence-based interventions for students who exhibit antisocial behavior patterns is a challenge that confronts our schools at every grade level. Many at-risk students have serious school adjustment problems that demand significant administrative time, disrupt regular classroom instruction, fail to respond to traditional school discipline practices, and, in some cases, pose a serious threat to the safety of other students or school staff. When not in school, these students often lack adult supervision and affiliate with other at-risk peers—circumstances that can easily lead to their involvement in juvenile crime.

RISK AND PROTECTIVE FACTORS

Boys and girls who engage in antisocial and potentially violent behavior in school have chronic and complex support needs. These students often experience multiple risk factors known to predict life-course juvenile delinquency, such as poverty, early aggression, family conflict, school failure, and high-crime neighborhoods (Loeber & Hay,

Vicki Nishioka, PhD, Institute on Violence and Destructive Behavior, College of Education, University of Oregon, Eugene, Oregon.

152

1997; Resnick et al., 1997; Smith & Carlson, 1997; Stoiber & Good, 1998). These universal risk factors span multiple domains of students' lives, disrupting relationships with their families, schools, peers, and communities. Frequently, at-risk students have few protective factors (i.e., effective parenting, adult mentoring relationship, associations with typical peers, and a strong school bond) to prevent or alter the escalating trajectory of antisocial behavior. As a result, these students often experience aggression, peer rejection, and learning difficulties during the early primary grades—school problems that persist throughout their school careers (Bullis, Walker, & Steiber, 1998; Kellam, Ling, Merisca, Brown, & Ialongo, 1998; Loeber & Farrington, 1998a; Wasserman & Miller, 1998). Table 7.1 lists the major risk and protective factors that influence the development of antisocial behavior patterns.

TABLE 7.1. Risk and Protective Factors for At-Risk Students

Risk factors	Protective factors
Individual	
• Early antisocial behavior • Impulsivity • Poor cognitive development • Peer rejection	• Self-control • Problem-solving skills • Competent interpersonal skills
Family	
• Ineffective parenting skills • High level of parent–child conflict • Parental antisocial behavior • Permissive parental attitudes toward antisocial behavior • Poverty	• Parental monitoring • Positive reinforcement • Positive parent–child communication • Limit setting • Effective parent–child problem solving
School	
• Low school engagement • Poor academic performance • Low school aspirations	• Positive relationship with an adult mentor • School engagement • Academic success
Peers	
• Association with deviant peers • Peer rejection	• Association with positive peer models • Recognition for positive participation and achievement • Opportunities for participation in healthy activities

Note. Adapted from Loeber, Green, Keenan, and Lahey (1995) and Dishion, French, and Patterson (1995).

GENDER DIFFERENCES

Although most risk and protective factors appear to be universal for both boys and girls, the literature suggests that there may be important gender differences that programs should consider. Girls that engage in aggressive behavior, like boys, are likely to have escalating patterns of school, peer, and family problems. However, girls have a higher prevalence of internalizing behaviors and tend to engage in more social or relational aggression rather than overt acting-out behavior (Leadbeater, Kuperminc, Blatt, & Hertzog, 1999). Social aggression includes acts such as giving "dirty looks," social manipulation, spreading malicious rumors, or withdrawal of friendship (Crick, Casas, & Mosher, 1997). Gender is a mediating factor in peer reactions to social aggression. Girls who engage in social aggression experience rejection by most peers. However, boys who show the same behavior may receive increased acceptance from some peers and rejection from others (Crick, Casas, & Mosher, 1997; Harrington, Rutter, & Fombonne, 1996; Huesmann & Guerra, 1997). Furthermore, boys and girls have different perceptions of social aggression. Boys view physical aggression as more hurtful than social aggression, whereas girls view social and physical aggression as equally hurtful (Galen & Underwood, 1997). Gender differences in the perception and expression of aggressive behavior may have important implications for screening of, and effective intervention with, female students.

Gender may also affect the relative value and importance of protective factors. Browne and Rife (1991) found that at-risk girls were more positive toward school than their male counterparts and tended to have stronger academic skills that might delay the onset of school problems. Protective factors identified as highly important to girls include school attachment, positive parent relationship, personal safety, and having an adult mentor (Leadbeater et al., 1999; Vance, Fernandez, & Biber, 1998).

The presence of multiple risk factors paired with limited support makes additional school services such as social skills training, adult mentoring, and positive behavior interventions essential for at-risk students. In addition, a portion of these students will require resources that extend beyond school-based services to the need for family interventions and linkages to community agencies.

The remainder of this chapter describes (1) features of successful alternative programs or classrooms; (2) targeted and indicated interventions that have proven effectiveness in promoting one or more protective factors; (3) multicomponent interventions that show promise in attaining long-term positive outcomes for at-risk students; and (4) family and community collaboration. This chapter also includes descriptions of effective and promising programs that illustrate one or more features of successful alternative programs. The selected interventions have (1) proven effectiveness through randomized clinical studies, (2) manualized procedures that allow replication, and (3) are school-based. The interventions described in this chapter, although noteworthy, by no means represent the full spectrum of effective programs. Box 7.1 contains a listing of resources regarding evidence-based programs.

BOX 7.1. Information Resources for Effective Interventions

- Derzon, J., Wilson, S. J., & Cunningham, C. (2001). *The effectiveness of school-based interventions for prevention and reduction of violence.* Washington, DC: George Washington University, Hamilton Fish Institute. *http://hamfish.org*

- Fashola, O. S., & Slavin, R. E. (1997). *Effective and replicable programs for students placed at risk in elementary and middle schools.* Washington, DC: U.S. Department of Education, Office of Educational Research and Improvement. *www.successforall.com/resource/research/effective.htm*

- Greenberg, M. T., Domitrovich, C., & Bumbarger, B. (1999). *Preventing mental disorders in school-age children: A review of the effectiveness of prevention programs.* University Park, PA: Pennsylvania State University, Prevention Research Center for the Promotion of Human Development. *www.prevention.psu.edu/pubs/CMHS.html*

- Mihalic, S., Irwin, K., Elliott, D., Fagan, A., & Hansen, D. (2001). *Blueprints for violence prevention* (OJJDP Juvenile Justice Bulletin). Washington DC: U.S. Department of Justice, Office of Justice Programs, Office of Juvenile Justice and Delinquency Prevention. *www.ncjrs.org/html/ojjdp/jjbul2001_7_3/contents.html*

- Center for Substance Abuse Prevention: Western Center. (2003). *Building a successful prevention program.* Reno: University of Nevada. *http://casat.unr.edu/westcapt/bestpractices/index.htm*

FEATURES OF SUCCESSFUL PROGRAMS AND SERVICES

Programs and services for at-risk students, often referred to as alternative education, vary greatly in their goals, organizational structures, and desired outcomes. Most programs respond to local needs, available funding, politics, and the prevailing school culture. Students may attend by choice, referral, or requirement. Settings may be a separate site, a "school within a school," or a self-contained classroom (Raywid, 1990). Little research exists comparing the relative effectiveness of these different program models (Tobin & Sprague, 2000). However, evaluations of targeted and selected interventions for at-risk students indicate that a number of evidence-based school and family interventions are available.

Tobin and Sprague (2000) reviewed effective school-based practices for students with behavior disorders and/or antisocial behavior, and recommended that these practices be combined to create an effective alternative education program. Interventions reviewed had proven results with students at-risk for antisocial behavior or failure in regular education and were practical for pubic school settings. Table 7.2 lists features common to these successful programs. In general, these features can be organized into four categories: (1) program structure and behavioral interventions, (2) mentoring and individualized case management, (3) social skills training and academic instruction, and (4) family and community collaboration.

Program Structure and Behavioral Interventions

Successful interventions or alternative classrooms for at-risk students provide services to smaller groups of students in highly organized settings that emphasize positive behavior support. Features of highly organized programs include (1) low ratio of students to teachers and informal interactions, (2) highly structured classrooms with positive behavior management, (3) a positive rather than punitive emphasis on behavior management, (4) individualized behavior support, and (5) functional behavioral assessment procedures. A description of these features follows:

Low Ratio of Students to Teachers and Informal Interactions

A common feature of successful alternative programs is a low student-to-staff ratio that encourages more personal staff time for students. Peterson, Bennet, and Sherman (1991) conducted qualitative interviews of uncommonly successful teachers of at-risk students nominated by administrators, teachers, and program directors. The teachers in this study identified building strong relationships with students and creating a "place of belonging and identity" as important features of successful teaching. Unlike traditional classrooms, teachers interrupted academic work to respond quickly to student problems and actively coached students to increase their success in social situations.

The Skills for Success program (Sprague, Walker, Nishioka, et al., 2001) provided services to at-risk students by using a "school within a school" approach. That is, the alternative classroom was housed in a public middle school setting as opposed to an off-site location. Students in this program attended regular classes for part or most of their school day to allow opportunities to socialize with typical peers. To ensure that students had personalized adult support, the teachers in this program used a morning "check-in" ritual to welcome students to school. Students were required to check in with alternative program staff before school started; there they also could enjoy hot chocolate and a light breakfast with other students. This morning ritual gave students the opportunity to plan for the school day and to request help for special assignments. If needed, students were also required to check out with alternative program staff at the end of the school day. These periods of "touching base" also gave students an opportunity to share home, peer, and community concerns that could affect their behavior in school. These discussions alerted staff to potential problem situations that required interventions to avoid their escalation into full-blown problems. Finally, these

TABLE 7.2. Features of Comprehensive Intervention Programs

Program structure and behavioral interventions

Highly structured classroom with positive behavior management
- Level systems provide predictable structure
- Self-management skills are taught
- High rates of positive reinforcement are delivered
- Extra academic support is provided
- Students are able to move to less restrictive settings

Positive rather than punitive emphasis on behavior management
- Rewards for acceptable behavior and compliance
- Directly teach clear classroom rules
- Begin with rich reinforcement and then "fade" to normal levels, when possible (four positives to one negative)

Individualized behavioral interventions based on functional assessment
- Identify causes of the behavior
- Identify what is "keeping it going"
- Identify positive behaviors to replace problems
- Interview and involve the student
- Use multicomponent interventions

Mentoring and informal interactions

Low ratio of students to teachers
- More personal time for each student
- Better behavioral gains
- Higher quality of instruction

Adult mentors at the school
- Mentor must use positive reinforcement
- Mentor takes special interest in student
- Mentor tracks behavior, attendance, attitude, grades
- Mentor negotiates alternative to suspension and expulsion

Social skills training and academic instruction

Social skills instruction
- Problem solving
- Conflict resolution
- Anger management
- Empathy for others

High-quality academic instruction
- Direct instruction plus learning strategies
- Control for difficulty of instruction
- Small, interactive groups
- Directed responses and questions of students

(continued)

TABLE 7.2. (*continued*)

- Service Learning
- Multicomponent school programs

<u>Family and community collaboration</u>

Involving parents
- Frequent home–school communication
- Parent education programs, provided either at school or in the community

Wraparound services
- Linkage to community services
- Coordinated service system

---

check-in/check-out times allowed staff to monitor students before and after school—periods that often had limited adult supervision.

Highly Structured Classroom with Positive Behavior Management

Positive classroom management reduces classroom disruption so that more time can be devoted to academic teaching (Wang, Haertel, & Walberg, 1994). Teachers of well-managed classrooms make sure students know and can perform the behavioral expectations for the classroom and school. Ideally, the classroom rules (1) are limited to three to five in number, (2) reflect the schoolwide rules, (3) positively state the desired behaviors, and (4) are clearly visible for all students (Colvin, Kame'enui, & Sugai, 1993; Walker et al., 1996). Students should also be taught classroom routines and social skills that will help them to follow rules, ask for help, and gain positive adult recognition (Levin & Ornstein, 1989; Wang, Oates, & Weishew, 1995). Effective classroom teachers give reminders and rewards to help students follow classroom rules (Levin & Ornstein, 1989). Teachers can remind students of hallway expectations, routines to get ready for class, and expectations in the lunchroom before they transition to other school settings or activities. Likewise, the routine of reviewing students' behavioral performances after completion of an activity can act as an incentive to participate.

Positive Rather Than Punitive Emphasis on Behavior Management

Classroom organization and behavior management systems that provide opportunities to teach and practice self-management and social skills are important prevention strategies for students at risk for chronic problem behaviors (Hudley & Graham, 1992; Nelson, Smith, Young, & Dodd, 1991). Positive behavioral interventions for these students reward positive behavioral choices, prevent students from gaining rewards from use of problem or antisocial behavior, and teach them specific social behaviors that they should use in place of problem behaviors. For example, the Skills for Success program uses a simple point system to monitor student behavior, academic engagement, and compliance with school rules in the alternative classroom. Teachers helped the students select an individual goal, self-assess or rate their behavior for each goal, and accept positive or negative behavioral consequences for their behavioral choices. At the end of each class, students self-assessed their behavior and classroom work during the preceding class period. Program staff then praised students for correct self-assessment and/or clarified behavior expectations for inaccurate self-assessment. Students earned free time, special privileges, and tangible rewards for achieving behavioral goals (Sprague, Walker, Nishioka, et al., 2001).

Individualized Positive Behavior Support

Many at-risk students start their aggressive behavior at a young age and, over the years, have learned how to disrupt, defy, and disobey teachers at a high level of proficiency. Unfortunately, traditional school sanctions such as detention, suspension, or verbal reprimands have become commonplace for these students and no longer serve as a deterrent to their problem behaviors (Mayer, 1995). In fact, many students may increase aggressive and authority conflict behaviors to escape unwanted schoolwork, gain peer attention, and/or avoid difficult situations. Similarly, traditional school rewards such as good grades, positive peer relationships, teacher praise, or special rewards may not be valued or are unattainable by these students unless they receive specialized school support.

Nelson and Roberts (2000) observed the ongoing interactions between teachers and 99 students with high rates of disruptive behavior and 278 typical students. Observation results revealed that at-risk students displayed many of the same behavior problems as typical students. These behaviors included breaking known rules, refusing to follow directions, and disrupting the class. However, typical students generally stopped the problem behavior in response to traditional school and classroom consequences. In contrast, at-risk students were extremely resistant to stopping problem behaviors in response to these consequences and engaged in problem behaviors at a higher rate and level of intensity. Thus, behavioral interventions that emphasize *prevention* rather than reactive or aversive teacher responses may promote positive changes in these students' behavior at less cost in teacher stress, school resources, and student failure.

Effective behavioral intervention strategies that reduce students' antisocial behavior are available. The Good Behavior Game is a classroom-based prevention model intended to reduce both aggressive and shy behaviors in elementary school children. The classroom teacher assigns students to teams, with equal numbers of aggressive/disruptive and shy students assigned to each team. The teacher then monitors each team's behavior by tallying noncompliant behaviors on the chalkboard. Teams not exceeding four tally marks at the end of the "game period" receive tangible rewards (Dolan et al., 1993). A longitudinal, randomized study involving 500 first-grade students at 14 public schools in five communities indicated significant short- and long-term effects. The program reduced peer-nominated aggressive behavior for boys; however, girls did not show a significant reduction. In addition, boys who demonstrated the highest rates of aggression in the treatment group demonstrated significantly less aggression in sixth grade (Kellam et al., 1998).

Most students with serious antisocial behavior patterns require multicomponent interventions that target reduced student behavior and positive changes in their family, school, and peers to achieve maximum success (Kamps, Kravits, Rauch, Kamps, & Chung, 2000; Walker et al, 1996). *First Step to Success* is one such multicomponent early intervention program that uses universal screening procedures to identify kindergarten students who show early signs of antisocial behavior patterns. This intervention provides coaching for the teacher so that the student is taught classroom expectations and receives high levels of reinforcement and consistent behavioral responses. In addition, parents are taught strategies for supporting their child's school progress. The results of a randomized, controlled study found significant improvement in adaptive behavior, reduced maladaptive behavior, and reduced aggression for students receiving the intervention. In addition, students significantly improved their academic engagement time (Walker et al., 1998). Several studies have further documented the powerful effects of the First Step to Success intervention (Epstein & Walker, 2002; Golly, Sprague, Walker, Beard, & Gorham, 2000; Walker, 1998).

Functional Behavioral Assessment

The use of behavior support plans based on functional behavioral assessment information is a promising approach for building highly organized intervention strategies that reduce student misbehavior (Sprague & Horner, 1999; Sugai, Lewis-Palmer, & Hagan, 1998). Research indicates that students may use misbehavior to gain things they want or to avoid tasks, demands, and situations they do not want. Functional behavioral assessment is a process that (1) clearly defines the student's problem behavior, (2) identifies possible reasons or functions for the misbehavior, and (3) determines consequences that maintain the misbehavior. This process also lists consequences (e.g., adult responses, school consequences, peer reactions) that may help/encourage the student to maintain the behavior. Additional information to elicit that may help planning teams develop an individualized behavior intervention includes identification of meaningful rewards for the student, alternative skills the student might use to replace the problem behavior, and interventions that may be worth trying. The functional behavioral assessment process uses semistructured interviews of teachers, parents, and other staff, review of student records, and direct observation of the student to collect the needed information (Kern, Dunlap, Clarke, & Childs, 1994; Kearney & Tillotson, 1998). When possible, the student should participate in both the functional behavioral assessment process and the development of his or her intervention plan (Reed, Thomas, Sprague, & Horner, 1997).

Mentoring and Individualized Case Management

At-risk students are challenging to teach, discipline, and support. Their repertoire of school discipline problems encompasses a diverse array of antisocial behaviors that most teachers find difficult to manage. Some students are argumentative, defiant, disruptive, and encourage peers to act out with them. Others may act out in less overt ways by lying, stealing, and spreading malicious rumors about others (Loeber & Farrington, 1998a, 1998b). These behavior problems often emerge during the early elementary years and result in a pattern of repeated reprimands, exclusionary practices, and academic failure that follows the student from classroom to classroom and school year to school year (Goldstein, 1999; Mayer, 1995). Consequently, many at-risk students perceive school as aversive and teachers as nonsupportive. For these reasons, a mentoring and positive adult relationship is critical to building the "school connectedness" so necessary for educational success (Browne & Rife, 1991).

Adult Mentoring Relationship

McPartland and Nettles (1991) define mentoring as a sustained "one-to-one relationship between a caring adult and a child who needs support to achieve academic, career, social, or personal goals" (p. 588). Although community-based mentoring programs such as Big Brothers/Big Sisters are the most well known, school-based programs are emerging as viable options for at-risk students. Benefits of mentoring programs based in the school setting include decreased scheduling and coordinating problems that may interfere with mentoring appointments. School-based mentors report more supervision as well as increased opportunities to communicate and, if needed, advocate for the child with his or her teacher(s) (Herrera, 1999; Herrera, Sipe, & McClanahan, 2000). Mentoring has multiple benefits for at-risk students, including (1) reductions in antisocial behavior, (2) decreased drug and alcohol use, and (3) improved school engagement, evidenced by better grades, attendance, and positive attitudes toward school (Beier, Rosenfeld, Spitalny, Zansky, & Bontempo, 2000; Sipe, 1996). Mentoring also helps build better relationships between the at-risk student and his or her teachers, parents, and peers (Grossman & Garry, 1997).

Critical features of successful mentoring programs include (1) clear goals that guide the program and each mentoring relationship; (2) careful matching of the mentor to the student to ensure shared interests and compatibility; (3) six or more hours of "prematch" training for the mentor, with ongoing monthly supervision; and (4) a high level of contact between mentor and student (three or more times per month) that includes social as well as academic activities (Grossman & Garry, 1997; Herrera et al., 2000).

Aim High is one example of a school-based mentoring program that recruited college students to mentor seventh- and eight-grade middle school students with antisocial behavior problems, a 2.0 or lower grade-point average, and at least one failing grade. Mentors' primary mission was to provide academic assistance in problematic subject areas and to serve as a positive role models for the students. Mentors met at least 1 hour per week throughout a semester with assigned students. Students who received mentoring significantly improved in the number of expulsions and severity of office discipline referrals when compared to students who did not receive mentoring. Mentored students also improved on social self-concept and social competence scales (Newton, 1994).

Individualized Case Management

Unfortunately, many students experience chronic adverse life events that interfere with their ability to accommodate the demands of schooling (Chung & Elias, 1996). Such events may include moving, family separations, financial difficulties, problems with peers, an arrest for a community-based crime, severe problems with a given teacher, or a family disruption. Frequently, these adverse events are unpredictable and may change the intensity as well as type of services the student requires. For this and other reasons, these students require repeated assessment of their risk status and case management of their service.

The teacher or lead staff person often fulfills several roles with the student and his or her family, including that of case manager. This professional (1) reinforces the student's positive efforts and achievements, (2) arranges meaningful and effective consequences for student misbehavior, and (3) ensures that instruction is important and relevant. Equally important, he or she provides collegial support and coaching to help regular classroom teachers avoid burnout or discouraged reactions to the student's intense behavioral and educational needs. In general, the teacher or school counselor is best-suited to case manage those students who require extensive parent communication, family support, and/or agency coordination. In contrast, students who require only school-based services may do well with a teacher's assistant, general education classroom teacher, or adult volunteer as their assigned case manager.

The case manager meets at least weekly and (for some students) as often as daily with his or her assigned student(s) to foster a positive mentoring relationship. During these meetings, the case manager provides guidance for the student by coaching him or her to make positive behavior changes in school, monitors the student's behavior and academic performance, and, most importantly, provides the support and presence of a trusted adult at school.

A successful school-based mentoring program, Check and Connect, provides at-risk students with a daily check-in and monitoring system to prevent dropout (Evelo, Sinclair, Hurley, Christenson, & Thurlow, 1996). The Check and Connect program organizes a simple student monitoring system, provides strategies for early detection of school problems, and suggests strategies for helping the student reconnect with schooling before failure and dropout occurs. The results of this targeted intervention for 363 elementary school students indicate that the percentage of students arriving to school on time increased from 42% at time of referral to 86% after 2 years of Check and Connect. In addition, the percentage of students who maintained 95% attendance rates more than doubled from 17% at referral to 40% at the 2-year mark. The results of a 5-year follow-along study for behaviorally at-risk high school students were equally promising. After 2 or more years, students placed in the Check and Connect intervention were more likely to be in school (48/70, or 68%) and were within 1 year of high school completion (27/70, or 38%). At the same point in time, 32/79 (41%) of the students in the control group were in school and 20/79 (25%) were within 1 year of graduation.

Social Skills Training and Academic Instruction

Students who have problems with antisocial behavior also have social and academic skills deficits that hinder their success in school and peer relationships. Many have difficulty with self-control, problem solving, and basic communication skills with peers and adults (Dumas, Blechman, & Prinz, 1994; Stanley, Dai, & Nolan, 1997; Walker & Leister, 1994). Moreover, these students often misinterpret the intentions of others, responding aggressively to perceived negative feedback or rejection, and they often lack the necessary skills to recruit and sustain social support networks (Rosenthal & Simeonsson, 1991). Consequently, poor interpersonal relationships, teacher and peer rejection, and family conflict are the common outcomes for at-risk students that contribute to an escalating pattern of antisocial behavior (Coie, Lochman, Terry & Hyman, 1992; Dishion, French, & Patterson, 1995).

Social Skills Training

A number of evidence-based social skills curriculum for students in kindergarten through high school are available. Most of these curriculum packages address skill building in self-control, problem solving, and anger management as well as specific coping strategies to replace the use of aggressive behaviors in difficult social situations. The majority of programs are designed for instruction in small-group situations (four to six students) that use role plays and activities to encourage active student participation.

Available social skills curricula vary considerably in design features such as target student population, length and frequency of sessions or lessons, follow-up or review sessions, and structured practice opportunities. Some social skills curricula are taught within a short time period, whereas others include follow-up or booster sessions to help students maintain skills. Curricula developed in recent years are designed to teach students across longer time periods—some, across multiple years—and include developmentally appropriate skill development in their training. In general, social skills curricula, delivered as the only intervention for the at-risk student, may produce immediate reduction of antisocial behavior but may not sustain the behavior change over time (Greenberg, Domitrovich, & Bumbarger, 1999; Mathur, Kavale, Quinn,

Forness, & Rutherford, 1998). One of the greatest challenges for schools serving at-risk students is to develop interventions that produce positive and sustainable behavior changes that, in turn, prevent the negative effects associated with antisocial behavior. Examples of each type of evidence-based social skills curriculum follow.

- The Anger Coping Program (Lochman, Burch, Curry, & Lampron, 1984) taught self-management, self-monitoring, perspective taking, and social problem-solving skills to small groups (four to six boys) of aggressive boys ages 9–12 years. The boys attended 12 weekly sessions taught by two adult coleaders. This indicated intervention showed significant reductions in the boys' aggressive behavior in both home and school settings as compared to boys who did not participate in the social skills training. In addition, boys who received the curriculum viewed themselves as more competent than boys in comparison groups. At 3 years following the intervention, 32 boys who participated in the program showed lower rates of drug and alcohol use and higher levels of self-esteem and social problem-solving skills. However, the long-term effects on delinquency rates and classroom behavior were not significant, although boys who received booster training did show some behavior improvement.

- The Social Relations Program was developed by Lochman, Coie, Underwood, and Terry (1993), leading researchers in the area of children's friendships and peer relationships. This social skills curriculum spans a longer time period: 26 weekly training sessions, designed to teach elementary school children to use problem-solving and anger coping skills to reduce aggressive responses to interpersonal conflicts. Teachers or counselors instruct students individually or in small groups. An evaluation of the program's impact on African American children (n = 52), ages 9–11 years, found that the children participating in the program were rated as significantly less aggressive by teachers and more socially accepted by peers at posttest than children in the control group. The effects of the intervention were maintained at 1-year follow-up.

- The I Can Problem Solve (ICPS) program is a social skills curriculum that begins in kindergarten and continues until early adolescence. ICPS teaches children how to think of nonviolent ways to solve everyday problems. The program has proven effectiveness in helping children learn to resolve interpersonal problems by using alternative social behaviors to replace aggression. This curriculum combines pictures, group interaction, and role-playing activities in 45 lessons that instructors teach to small groups of 6–10 children. The ICPS is available at three developmental levels: preschool, kindergarten and primary grades, and intermediate elementary grades. Students taught the curriculum demonstrated less impulsive and inhibited classroom behavior as well as better problem-solving skills compared to students in the control group (Shure & Spivac, 1980). Those children who received training and were most improved in the problem-solving skills were also the most improved in observed behaviors. Importantly, youngsters not showing behavior problems in preschool were less likely to begin showing them later. At the end of the school year, 71% of the trained students were rated as adjusted, compared to 54% of the students in the control group.

Furthermore, the ratings of impulsive and inhibited children increased from "adjust-ed" to higher reduction in problem behaviors of the 113 trained pre-kindergarten and kindergarten inner-city children compared to the 106 children in the control group.

High-Quality Academic Instruction

Selection of relevant and evidence-based curricula is essential to promoting successful learning for at-risk students (Tobin & Sprague, 2000). Classroom programs that con-nect academic curriculum to the lives and experiences of at-risk students may produce stronger academic outcomes. Of equal importance is the use of evidence-based instructional strategies that engage students in positive learning experiences (Coble & Piscatelli, 2002). Characteristics of effective classroom management include (1) high rates of interaction between the teacher and students, (2) the encouragement of higher thinking skills, (3) use of teaching strategies that actively engage students in their own learning, and (4) emphasis on language and literacy development (Levin & Ornstein, 1989; Martens & Kelly, 1993; Waxman & Huang, 1997). Teaching strategies that have demonstrated success with disadvantaged students include direct instruction, peer tutoring, cooperative learning, and service learning (Franca, Kerr, Reitz, & Lambert, 1990; Lloyd, Forness, & Kavale, 1998; Stevens & Slavin, 1995).

The Seattle Social Development Project (Hawkins et al., 1992), for example, is a multidimensional intervention that has a strong emphasis on increasing effective teaching practices. Teachers receive extensive training in positive classroom manage-ment, interactive teaching, and cooperative learning. First- and sixth-grade teachers also teach students important social behaviors that increase effective problem solving, positive peer relationships, and refusal skills. Parents receive training in family man-agement, supporting their children's academic progress, and encouraging positive relationships with peers.

Evaluation of the Seattle Social Development Project indicates improved school performance, school engagement, and family relationships, reduced antisocial behav-ior, and lower alcohol and delinquency problems in later grades (Hawkins et al., 1992). To assess the effects of full intervention and late intervention, researchers conducted a nonrandomized controlled trial with three conditions: (1) the full-inter-vention group received the intervention package from grades 1–6; (2) the late-inter-vention group received the intervention package in grades 5 and 6 only; and (3) the control group received no special intervention. After 6 years of the intervention, researchers collected information from 598 18-year-old students. Those who had been in the full-intervention group reported stronger attachment to school, self-reported improvement in achievement, and less involvement in school misbe-havior than did controls (Hawkins, Von Cleve, & Catalano, 1991; Hawkins, Catalano, Kosterman, Abbott, & Hill, 1999). There were no significant effects for the full- or late-intervention groups in lifetime prevalence of cigarette, alcohol, marijuana, or other illicit drug use at age 18. However, significant effects were found in the number of full-intervention participants who had committed violent acts, reported heavy alcohol use in the past year, or engaged in sexual intercourse, when compared to control group participants.

Service Learning

Service Learning is a promising intervention for at-risk students that integrates academic curricula and practical experience via community service activities and student reflection to increase school attachment, attendance, grades, and awareness of civic responsibility. This teaching strategy requires a high level of interaction between students and teacher, involves students in higher thinking skills, and connects academic curricula to the relevant issues in their community. Students who participate in Service Learning projects (1) identify and research a community need or problem, (2) use problem-solving skills to plan a service project that will address the need or problem, (3) participate in the community service activity, and (4) are encouraged to reflect upon the personal and community impact of the project (Boston, 1998). A national evaluation of Service Learning programs showed a reduction in juvenile arrests and teenage pregnancies for middle school students. There is also evidence that Service Learning increases skills in self-awareness, motivation, empathy, and communication for at-risk students (ABT Associates, 1998; Frey, 2003; Poole, 1997).

Multicomponent School Programs

In the simplest terms, the primary educational goal for antisocial students is to provide early intervention and prevention services that will help them achieve sustained success in school, at home, and in the community. There is a growing consensus that schools need to provide highly organized multicomponent interventions (Gottfredson, 2001). For most at-risk students, multicomponent interventions should begin early, continue through middle and high school, and target the range of risk and protective factors rather than isolated behavior (Greenberg et al., 1999; Walker et al., 1996). Additionally, interventions that encourage parent involvement, positive changes in family functioning, and linkages to the student's community may result in stronger long-term effects.

Problems with Grouping Antisocial Students

An important consideration for schools is the potential risks and benefits that arise from grouping at-risk students in one program. Such programs that serve at-risk students strategically organize use of group interventions to prevent unwanted problems, such as *increased* antisocial behavior and linkages to deviant peers when these students are placed in the same setting (Dishion & Andrews, 1995). One strategy to buffer possible problems with grouping antisocial students is the use of careful screening to ensure that the program accepts only those students who have problems or deficits targeted by the intervention (Reid, 1991). In addition, programs should avoid isolating at-risk students from their typical peers; indeed the programs should provide maximum opportunities for these youth to participate in positive activities with typical peers. Finally, the selected interventions should be highly organized, implemented with fidelity, and have proven effectiveness with the targeted population.

The Fast Track program, for example, provides comprehensive selected and indicated interventions for at-risk students in grades K–10. In the early grades, at-risk students are involved in social skills groups and activities. However, in grades 6–10, program developers limit group interventions to highly structured and brief orientation activities with parents and students to prevent socialization between at-risk students. The Fast Track intervention includes six components: (1) schoolwide instruction in the Promoting Alternative Thinking Strategies (PATHS) curriculum, (2) parent training groups, (3) home visits to assist the parents in problem solving, self-efficacy, and life management, (4) target social skills groups, (5) student tutoring in reading, and (6) peer pairing to enhance students' relationships with typical peers. Students also receive individualized services matched to their specific needs (e.g., tutoring, mentoring, family problem solving, and linkage to community agencies; Conduct Problems Prevention Research Group, 1992).

In one Fast Track program evaluation, 891 high-risk first-grade boys and girls were randomly assigned to two groups: 445 students were placed in the Fast Track group, and 446 students were placed in the no-intervention group. Evaluation results indicated positive outcomes for Fast Track students sustained across time. Overall, students showed less aggressive behavior in school and at home. As adolescents, the intervention group had lower percentages of arrests. Fast Track students also demonstrated increases in social and academic skills as compared to the control group. Moreover, their parents forced more consistent discipline, had higher involvement with their child, and reported greater satisfaction than parents of students who did not receive services. After 4 years of Fast Track services, teacher ratings, parent ratings, peer nominations, and self-report measures showed student improvement in the area of conduct problems, increased acceptance by peers, and reduced affiliation with deviant peers (Conduct Problems Prevention Research Group, 1999).

Reconnecting Youth is an intervention that targets students in grades 9–12 who have multiple problem behaviors such as aggression, substance abuse, depression, and poor school engagement. Students attend daily classes to learn social skills strategies that will increase their self-esteem, decision-making, self-control, and interpersonal communication skills. Classes are limited to 10–12 students and meet for one semester or 80 sessions. Other program components include student participation in structured activities during school and nonschool hours, increased parent involvement, and procedures to assist student crisis situations. Students who complete this intervention demonstrate improved grades, reduced drug use, and decreased problems with aggression, as compared to students who do not receive the training (Eggert, Thompson, Pike, & Randell, 2002; Eggert, Thompson, Herting, & Randell, 2001).

Family and Community Collaboration

The importance of parent involvement and effective parenting as a protective factor for students who engage in antisocial behavior is well documented (Kazdin, 1997; Loeber, Green, Keenan, & Lahey, 1995; Smith & Stern, 1997; Tiet et al., 1998). Family factors that increase children's resilience include positive attachment to at least one parent, consistent parenting, and effective supervision (Cauce, Felner, & Primavera, 1982; Smith & Carlson, 1997). In contrast, at-risk students experience high rates of parent–child conflict, harsh discipline, neglect, family disorganization, and ineffective parenting (Dishion, French, & Patterson, 1995; Ramsey & Walker, 1988). Furthermore, the negative impact of poor family functioning on student's behavior, peer acceptance, and academic success appear to occur regardless of gender, ethnic background, or age group (Arbona, Jackson, McCoy, & Blakely, 1999; Henggeler, Edwards, & Borduin, 1987; Stanger, Achenbach, & McConaughy, 1993). Finally, the chronic pattern of adverse life events and daily hassles that often challenges at-risk students and their families may increase parental stress to the point that parenting becomes ineffective (Ge, Conger, Lorenz, & Simons, 1994; Shaw, Winslow, Owens, & Hood, 1998; Tiet et al., 1998; Tolan, 1988).

Parent Involvement with the School

There is substantial evidence that parents' involvement in their children's schools has significant impact on the academic success of all students, including disadvantaged and at-risk populations (Christenson & Christenson, 1998; Henderson & Berla, 1994; Miedel & Reynolds, 1999). *Parent involvement* encompasses a variety of activities, such as:

- Attendance at school events, parent conferences, and scheduled meetings
- Quality home–school communication about student progress and programs
- Home learning activities (e.g., parents reading with their children; visiting educational resources)
- Family schedules that include an established time to do homework and reduced television viewing
- Volunteering to help with school activities or governance (Cotton & Wikelund, 1989; Epstein, 1992; Chavkin & Williams, 1993)

Typical school efforts to increase parent involvement include parent–teacher communication, school newsletters, school-sponsored family events, making available a variety of parent-volunteer opportunities, and including parents on school governance committees. Not surprisingly, these traditional school efforts have limited success with parents of at-risk students due to educational, cultural, and social barriers (Lareau,

1987). For example, parents of disadvantaged students tend to have lower educational backgrounds and, in many instances, had difficulty in school themselves. Consequently, these parents often have lower academic expectations of their child and provide limited home-learning activities. In addition, parents may perceive the role of schools and family as discrete and assign primary responsibility for their child's education to the school. Finally, limited transportation, time constraints, and language barriers prevent school involvement for some parents.

The contribution of poor parent involvement and ineffective parenting to the antisocial behavior and subsequent academic failure of at-risk students suggests that inclusion of strategies that improve parent involvement is critically important to student success—especially for younger students (Walker, Ramsey, & Gresham, 2004). For example, the High Scope Perry Preschool Project used active learning strategies to teach students considered high risk for school failure to be active learners (Weikart, Rogers, Adcock, & McClelland, 1971). The teacher received extensive training in classroom organization and teaching strategies that promoted active, student-directed learning that spanned math, science, reading, art, music, social studies, and movement. In addition, parents were invited to attend a monthly group meeting to encourage their positive support and school involvement.

Evaluation of the High Scope Perry Preschool project showed immediate short-term gains in academic outcomes that were not maintained in elementary school. However, longitudinal studies have found significant and sustained behavioral outcomes, including lower rates of crime and delinquency, teenage pregnancy, and welfare dependency (Schweinhart, Barnes, & Weikart, 1993). Moreover, youth also demonstrated higher rates of academic achievement, employment, positive social relationships, and family stability as young adults.

Parent Training

Ineffective parenting is considered a strong predictor of social maladjustment and antisocial behaviors for at-risk students (Dishion et al., 1995). Successful parent-training models teach parents problem-solving skills, communication, relationship building, and disciplinary skills that are individualized to reflect the specialized needs and circumstances of the at-risk student and his or her family (Thompson, Ruma, Schuchmann, & Burks, 1995). Factors that increase and maintain participation in parent-training classes include the use of experienced trainers perceived as helpful by participating parents. These trainers use humor and warmth to create a nurturing setting (Diamond, Serrano, Dickey, & Sonis, 1996). Furthermore, parent trainers who are attentive to parent response and use nonconfrontational approaches appear to have greater success with parents of at-risk students.

The Adolescent Transitions Program (ATP) is a curriculum that targets instruction in five parenting skills that have proven effectiveness with youth who engage in antisocial behavior (Dishion & Andrews, 1995): effective parental monitoring, positive rein-forcement, parent–child communications, limit setting, and problem solving. Irvine and colleagues (Irvine, Biglan, Smolkowski, Metzler, & Ary, 1999) evaluated the effec-tiveness of the ATP using group leaders who had little-to-no prior experience in parent training. The results of this study showed improved problem solving between parent and child, increased consistency in parent discipline, and a reduction in the adolescents' antisocial behavior problems.

Parent-training programs also have demonstrated effectiveness with at-risk stu-dents from diverse ethnic backgrounds. Family Effectiveness Training is designed to serve Hispanic families with 6- to 12-year-old children who have problems with antisocial behavior, associate with deviant peers, and have frequent conflict with their parents. This intervention uses structured family discussion and activities to help parents improve their family management skills and to improve positive com-munication among family members. An evaluation of this intervention indicated sig-nificant reduction in children's contact with deviant peers, decreased antisocial behavior, and marked improvement in family functioning (Szapocznik & Williams, 2000).

A major barrier to the effectiveness of parent-education programs is low participa-tion and completion rates. Kazdin's (1997) review of parent-training research found 40–60% of families that began treatment left the program early. Factors that were asso-ciated with this high attrition rate were low socioeconomic status, younger-age moth-ers, single-parent families, high levels of parental stress, poor social support, and a his-tory of parent delinquency. This high attrition rate has resulted in the development of creative alternatives to traditional parent-training programs.

The Parenting Wisely intervention teaches parents effective intervention strate-gies for substance abuse and antisocial behavior problems of their 9- to 18-year-old children. A unique feature of this program is the use of self-administered computer programs to conduct the training. This program provides information for parents in a nonjudgmental manner using highly interactive software. Parenting Wisely has been utilized by African American, Hispanic, and Caucasian families who generally do not seek out, or participate in, parent education or mental health treatment for their chil-dren's problems. A number of randomized studies indicated an increase in parent understanding of effective parenting skills, improved problem solving, and reduced use of physical punishment. In addition, statistically significant improvements in behavior were achieved for 20–55% of the children (Kacir & Gordon, 1997; Segal, Chen, Kacir, & Gyglys, 2003).

Family Management

The development of multicomponent family interventions responds to the assumption that at-risk students and their families require support for multiple risk factors that negatively influence their stability and positive functioning. Moreover, programs that target positive skill development for the student in addition to effective strategies at home and school may achieve more positive and longer-lasting reductions in students' antisocial behavior (Greenberg et al., 1999).

The Linking the Interests of Families and Teachers (LIFT) program is a multicomponent intervention that targets positive changes in the student's home life, personal and social competence levels, classroom performance/behavior, and peer group relationships. LIFT teaches parents effective, home-based forms of discipline and supervision, including consistent limit setting and involvement. At school, students participate in a 20-session program to increase their communication and problem-solving skills, and the strategies they use to resist negative peer influences. Finally, LIFT uses a version of the Good Behavior Game (see pp. 159–160) to reduce inappropriate physical aggression on the playground. A randomized, controlled study of this intervention found reductions in playground aggression as well as improved family problem solving (Eddy, Reid, & Fetrow, 2000; Reid, Eddy, Fetrow, & Stoolmiller, 1999). In addition, 30 months following completion of LIFT, students in the treatment group had significantly fewer arrests than those students who did not participate in LIFT.

Community Linkage and Family Support

The demands of children and youth who display antisocial behavior can overwhelm many parents. In addition to antisocial behavior patterns, at-risk students typically have a range of other concerns such as learning disorders, mental health disorders, alcohol and substance abuse problems, strained family relationships, homelessness, and/or teen parenting responsibilities. Many at-risk students have multiple problems at serious levels, making it unrealistic to expect a single intervention to address the heterogeneous needs of this population.

Students with multiple and complex service needs may require a case manager to collaborate with community social service agencies. The purpose of service coordination is to build linkages to community agencies that can ensure the fulfillment of the student's basic needs (e.g., food, safety, urgent medical/dental, clothing). Case managers work collaboratively with families, schools, and community agencies (1) to identify the needs of the student and his or her family, (2) to identify natural and agency supports that might be helpful, and (3) to coordinate services so that families receive timely and user-friendly forms of help (Eber, Nelson, & Miles, 1997). Burns, Farmer, Angold, Costello and Behar (1996) compared the efficacy of multiagency service teams led by a case manager versus a primary mental health clinician for students with serious emotional and behavior disorders. The results indicated that youth who had a designated case manager participated in services longer and used a wider variety of them.

Effective coordination of community services is difficult because of multiple systemic barriers. Rigid procedures, high caseloads, and inadequate resources often hinder agency workers. Family issues also contribute to poor coordination due to poor self-advocacy, distrust of agency and school staff, and purposeful avoidance of agency supervision. Taken together, these factors may create inefficient services that fail to help and, in some cases, may even hinder the student's progress. In these situations, the case manager may provide the organization, communication, and follow-through necessary to restore trust and productive relationships between the agency/agencies and family.

Early Risers: Skills for Success is a multicomponent program that serves 6- to 10-years-old children who display aggressive, disruptive, and/or uncooperative behaviors (August, Realmuto, Hektner, & Bloomquist, 2001). Children served by this program receive regular contact and support from an adult mentor or family advocate at school and in their home. Each family advocate serves a caseload of 25–30 child and family participants. During these mentoring visits, the family advocate provides recognition for the child as well as training in skills that will help him or her sustain positive family and peer relationships. In addition, the family advocate facilitates communication between the school and child's parents by providing consultation and support, as needed. This program also conducts regular parent and child groups that include both individual and combined activities between the child and parent. Finally, the advocate helps the family connect to community services such as Boy Scouts, Girl Scouts, YMCA, mental health, and human resources. The children who participated in this program showed improvement on academic and social skills as well as decreased aggressive behavior. Effects were significant for both boys and girls.

Multisystemic Therapy (MST) is another program that incorporates parent training, family management, and linkage to social service agencies for at-risk students. MST serves 12- to 17-year-old students who have problems with chronic antisocial and substance abuse behaviors. Youths served by this program have multiple arrests, associate with deviant peers, are failing in school, and have families with multiple needs. The primary goal of MST is to empower families so that they can use natural support systems to manage their needs. The MST therapist helps parents set reasonable goals, eliminate barriers that interfere with family stability, and increase effective parenting. A number of randomized clinical studies of this intervention indicate that MST significantly reduces substance use and antisocial behavior for program youth; subsequent 2- and 4-year follow-up studies indicate that these positive changes are sustained over time (Henggeler, Mihalic, Rone, Thomas, & Timmons-Mitchell, 1998).

Table 7.3 summarizes these evidence-based programs.

TABLE 7.3. Evidence-Based Program Examples Summary

Program	Authors/resource information	Type of intervention	Student characteristics
Functional Behavioral Assessment	Positive Behavior Interventions and Support *www.pbis.org*	Individual student behavior intervention	All ages with behavior disorders
Good Behavior Game	Kellam Sheppard, PhD American Institutes for Research *www.bpp.jhu.edu*	Classroom/school intervention	Grades K–10 students with conduct problems
Service Learning	National Service Learning Clearinghouse *www.servicelearning.org*	Group/classroom teaching strategy	All ages, ranging from typical to at risk
Anger Coping Program	Jim Larson, PhD John Lochman, PhD Therapeutic Resources *www.therapeuticresources.com*	Social skills training; small-group intervention with 18 weekly meetings	8- to 12-year-olds with aggression problems
I Can Problem Solve (ICPS)	Myrna Shure, PhD *www.thinkingchild.com*	Social skills training; whole-school/ multiyear prevention program	Preschool, elementary, and middle school students with aggression problems
Promoting Alternative Thinking Strategies (PATHS)	Carole Kursche, PhD Mark Greenberg, PhD Channing Bete Company *www.channingbete.com*	Social skills training; whole-school/ multiyear prevention program	Grades K–6 students
Social Relations Program	John E. Lochman, PhD John D. Coie, PhD University of Alabama *jlochman@gp.as.ua.edu*	Social skills training; small-group intervention with 26 weekly sessions	Grade 4 students with aggression and/ or peer rejection problems

(continued)

TABLE 7.3. (*continued*)

Program	Authors/resource information	Type of intervention	Student characteristics
Big Brothers/ Big Sisters	Big Brothers/Big Sisters *national@bbsa.org*	Mentoring; individual student intervention with recommended 1½- to 2-year time commitment	Students of all ages from single-parent homes
Check and Connect	David Evelo, MA Mary Sinclair, PhD Christine Hurley, PhD Sandra Christenson, PhD Martha Thurlow, PhD *ici.umn.edu/checkandconnect/*	Mentoring; individual student with recommended 2-year time commitment	Grades K–12 students at risk for school dropout
Adolescent Transitions Program (ATP)	Thomas J. Dishion, PhD Kate Kavanagh, PhD Child and Family Center *asimas@darkwing.uoregon.edu*	Multicomponent intervention; parent groups for 12 weekly sessions	Parents of 10- to 14-year-old youth at high risk for antisocial behavior
Family Effectiveness Training	José Szapocznik, PhD University of Miami School of Medicine, Center for Family Studies *www.cfs.med.miami.edu*	Family management training; 13 family sessions	Hispanic families with children ages 6–12 with behavior problems
Parenting Wisely	Don Gordon, PhD Family Works, Inc. *www.familyworksinc.com*	Parent training; interactive, computer-based training for individuals or small parent groups	Parents of 8- to 18-year-old youth at risk for delinquency or substance abuse
Early Risers: Skills for Success	Gerald J. August, PhD George M. Realmuto, PhD Michael L. Bloomquist, PhD University of Minnesota *Augus001@tc.umn.edu*	Multicomponent and multiyear program for individual students and families	Elementary school students ages 6–10; family advocates for students at risk for school failure

(*continued*)

TABLE 7.3. (*continued*)

Program	Authors/resource information	Type of intervention	Student characteristics
Fast Track	Conduct Problems Prevention Research Group *www.fasttrackproject.org*	Multicomponent and multiyear program for whole school	Elementary, middle, and high school students in disadvantaged neighborhoods
First Step to Success	Hill Walker, PhD Bruce Stiller, PhD Annemieke Golly, PhD Kathryn Kavanagh, PhD Herbert Severson, PhD Edward G. Feil, PhD Sopris West Publications *www.sopris.org*	Multicomponent program for individual students and parents	Grades K–2 students with aggressive behavior problems
Functional Family Therapy	James F. Alexander, PhD Department of Psychology University of Utah *www.ffinc.com*	Multicomponent program for individual students and families, with 12 weekly sessions	10- to 18-year-olds at risk for antisocial behavior and alcohol/drug use
High Scope Perry Preschool Project	David Wikert, PhD High/Scope Educational Research Foundation *www.highscope.org*	Multicomponent and multiyear project for preschool programs	3- to 4-year-olds at risk for school failure
Linking the Interests of Families and Teachers (LIFT)	John Reid, PhD Mark Eddy, PhD Rebecca Fastow, PhD *www.oslc.org/dproj.hrm/#lift*	Multicomponent and multiyear project for whole school	Grades 1–5 students
Multisystemic Therapy (MST)	Scott Henggler, PhD Multisystemic Therapy Services MST Services, Inc. *www.mstservices.com*	Multicomponent program for individual students and families: 1 therapist per 15 families per year	Juvenile offenders at risk for out-of-home placement

(*continued*)

TABLE 7.3. (*continued*)

Program	Authors/resource information	Type of intervention	Student characteristics
Seattle Social Development	J. David Hawkins, PhD Richard Catalano, PhD Seattle Development Research Group *www.depts.washington.edu/sdrg*	Multicomponent and multiyear program for whole school	Grades 1–5 students in disadvantaged neighborhoods

CONCLUSION

Students who engage in antisocial and potentially violent behavior present many challenges for schools. Typically, at-risk students experience early aggression that is highly resistant to change and that, without intervention, will continue to escalate throughout their school career. Successful intervention programs start early and continue to provide service into adolescence. A number of evidence-based strategies have proven effective in reducing antisocial behavior for at-risk students. These interventions range from single-component strategies that target a small cluster of skill and behavior gains to comprehensive, multicomponent programs that promote positive systemic changes toward the goal of long-term student success.

Despite these many successes, schools and social service agencies require more research to maximize their effectiveness with this challenging student population. There is evidence that gender, ethnicity, and developmental age differences may exist for at-risk students; however, the nature and impact of these differences on identification, prevention, and intervention strategies for this population remains in need of further investigation.

References

ABT Associates. (1998). *National evaluation of learn and serve school and community-based programs*. Washington, DC: Corporation for National Service.

Achenbach, T. (1991). *The Child Behavior Checklist: Manual for the teacher's report form*. Burlington, VT: Department of Psychiatry, University of Vermont.

American Psychological Association. (1993). *Violence and youth: Psychology's response: Vol. I. Summary report of the American Psychological Association's Commission on Violence and Youth*. Washington, DC: Author.

Arbona, C., Jackson, R. H., McCoy, A., & Blakely, C. (1999). Ethnic identity as a predictor of attitudes of adolescents toward fighting. *Journal of Early Adolescence, 19*, 323–340.

Association of California School Administrators. (1995). *Preventing chaos in times of crisis: A guide for administrators*. Sacramento, CA: Author.

August, G. J., Realmuto, G. M., Hektner, J. M., & Bloomquist, M. L. (2001). An integrated components preventive intervention for aggressive elementary school children: The Early Risers program. *Journal of Consulting and Clinical Psychology, 69*, 614–626.

Beier, S. R., Rosenfeld, W. D., Spitalny, K. C., Zansky, S. M., & Bontempo, A. N. (2000). The potential role of an adult mentor in influencing high-risk behaviors in adolescents. *Annals of Pediatric and Adolescent Medicine, 154*(4), 327–331.

Biglan, A. (1995). Translating what we know about the context of antisocial behavior into a lower prevalence of such behavior. *Journal of Applied Behavior Analysis, 28*, 479–492.

Biglan, A., Wang, M. C., & Walberg, H. J. (2003). *Preventing youth problems*. New York: Kluwer Academic/Plenum Publishers.

Boles, S., Biglan, A., & Smolkowski, K. (2003). *Relationships among negative and positive behaviors in adolescence*. Manuscript submitted for publication.

Boston, B. O. (1998). *Service-learning: What it offers to students, schools, and communities*. Washington, DC: Council of Chief State School Officers.

Bosworth, K., Espelage, D. L., & Simon, T. R. (1999). Factors associated with bullying behavior in middle school students. *Journal of Early Adolescence, 19*, 341–362.

Bronfenbrenner, U. (1979). *The ecology of human development: Experiments by nature and design*. Cambridge, MA: Harvard University Press.

Brophy, A. L. (1986). Confidence intervals for true scores and retest scores on clinical tests. *Journal of Clinical Psychology, 42*(6), 989–991.

Brophy, J., & Evertson, C. (1981). *Student characteristics and teaching*. New York: Longman.

Browne, C. S., & Rife, J. C. (1991). Social, personality, and gender differences in at-risk and not at-risk sixth grade students. *Journal of Early Adolescence, 11*, 482–495.

Bryk, A. S., & Driscoll, M. E. (1988). *The high school as community: Contextual influences and consequences for students and teachers*. Madison, WI: National Center on Effective Secondary Schools, Wisconsin Center for Education Research, University of Wisconsin–Madison.

Bullis, M., Walker, H. M., & Steiber, S. (1998). The influence of peer and educational variables on arrest status among at-risk males. *Journal of Early Adolescence, 11*, 482–495.

Burns, B. J., Farmer, E. M. Z., Angold, A., Costello, E. J., & Behar, L. (1996). A randomized trial of case management for youths with serious emotional disturbance. *Journal of Clinical Child Psychology, 25*, 476–486.

Burns, B., & Hoagwood, K. (2002). *Community treatment for youth: Evidence-based interventions for severe emotional and behavioral disorders*. New York: Oxford University Press.

Callaghan, S., & Joseph, S. (1995). Self-concept and peer victimization among school children. *Personality and Individual Differences, 18*, 161–163.

Cauce, A. M., Felner, R. D., & Primavera, J. (1982). Social support in high-risk adolescents: Structural components and adaptive impact. *American Journal of Community Psychology, 10*, 417–429.

Center for Substance Abuse Prevention: Western Center. Building a Successful Prevention Program. Reno, NV: University of Nevada. Available at *http://casat.unr.edu/westcapt/bestpractices/index.htm*

Chavkin, N. F., & Williams, D. L., Jr. (1993). Minority parents and the elementary school: Attitudes and practices. In N. Chavkin (Ed.), *Families and schools in a pluralistic society*. Albany, NY: State University of New York Press.

Christenson, S. L., & Christenson, J. C. (1998). *Family, school, and community influences on children's learning: A literature review* (Report No. 1, Live and Learn Project). Minneapolis: University of Minnesota Extension Service.

Chung, H., & Elias, M. (1996). Patterns of adolescent involvement in problem behaviors: Relationship to self-efficacy, social competence, and life events. *American Journal of Community Psychology, 24*, 771–785.

Coble, C. R., & Piscatelli, J. (2002). *Teaching quality: A national perspective*. Denver, CO: Education Commission of the States.

Coie, J. (1994, July 21). *The prevention of violence*. Keynote address presented at the OSEP Annual National Research Director's Conference. Washington, DC: U.S. Office of Special Education Programs.

Coie, J. D., Lochman, J. E., Terry, R., & Hyman, C. (1992). Predicting early adolescent disorder from childhood aggression and peer rejection. *Journal of Consulting Clinical Psychology, 60*, 783–792.

Colvin, G., Kame'enui, E. J., & Sugai, G. (1993). Reconceptualizing behavior management and school-wide discipline in general education. *Education and Treatment of Children, 16*, 361–381.

Colvin, G., Sugai, G., Good, R. H., III, & Lee, Y. (1997). Using active supervision and precorrection to improve transition behaviors in an elementary school. *School Psychology Quarterly, 12*(4), 344–363.

Committee for Children. (1993). *Second step: A violence prevention curriculum.* Seattle: Author.

Committee for Children. (2002). *Second step violence prevention curricula.* Seattle: Author.

Conduct Problems Prevention Research Group. (1992). A developmental and clinical model for the prevention of conduct disorder: The FAST Track Program. *Development and Psychopathology, 4,* 509–527.

Conduct Problems Prevention Research Group. (1999). Initial impact of the Fast Track prevention trial for conduct problems: I. The high-risk sample. *Journal of Consulting and Clinical Psychology, 67,* 631–647.

Cornell, D., & Sheras, P. (2003). *Threat assessment protocol.* Virginia Youth Violence Project, Curry School of Education, University of Virginia, Charlottesville, VA.

Cotton, K., & Wikelund, K. R. (1989). *Parent involvement in education.* In School Improvement Research Series III. Washington, DC: U.S. Department of Education, Office of Educational Research and Improvement (OERI). Available at: *www.nwrel.org/scpd/sirs/3/cu6.html.*

Craig, W. M., & Pepler, D. J. (1997). Observations of bullying and victimization in the schoolyard. *Canadian Journal of School Psychology, 13,* 41–59.

Crick, N. R., Casas, J. F., & Mosher, M. (1997). Relational and overt aggression in preschool. *Developmental Psychology, 33,* 579–588.

Crick, N. R., & Grotpeter, J. K. (1995). Relational aggression, gender, and social–psychological adjustment. *Child Development, 66,* 710–722.

Crone, D. A., & Horner, R. H. (2003). *Building positive behavior support systems in schools: Functional behavioral assessment.* New York: Guilford Press.

Crowe, T. (1991). *Habitual offenders: Guidelines for citizen action and public responses.* Washington, DC: Office of Juvenile Justice and Delinquency Prevention, U.S. Department of Justice.

Del'Homme, M., Kasari, C., Forness, S., & Bagley, R. (1996). Prereferral intervention and students at-risk for emotional and behavioral disorders. *Education and Treatment of Children, 19*(3), 272–285.

DeMary, J. L., Cox, H. D., Irby, G. H. Sr., & Cundiff, A. D. (2002). *Resource guide for crisis management in Virginia schools.* A. J. Atkinson & J. Anne (Eds.). Virginia Department of Education. Retrieved December 19, 2003, from *www.pen.k12.va.us/VDOE/Instruction/crisis-guide.pdf*

DeMary J. L., Owens, M., & Ramnarain, A. K. (2000). *School safety audit protocol.* Virginia Department of Education, Richmond, VA.

Derzon, J., Wilson, S. J., & Cunningham, C. (2001). *The effectiveness of school-based interventions for prevention and reduction of violence.* Washington, DC: George Washington University, Hamilton Fish Institute. Available at *http://hamfish.org*

Diamond, G. S., Serrano, A. C., Dickey, M., & Sonis, W. A. (1996). Current status of family-based outcome and process research. *Journal of the American Academy of Child and Adolescent Psychiatry, 35,* 6–17.

Dishion, T. J., & Andrews, D. W. (1995). Preventing escalation in problem behaviors with high-risk young adolescents: Immediate and 1-year outcomes. *Journal of Consulting and Clinical Psychology, 63,* 538–548.

Dishion, T. J., French, D. C., & Patterson, G. R. (1995). The development and ecology of antisocial behavior. In D. Cicchetti & D. J. Cohen (Eds.), *Developmental psychopathology. Vol. 2: Risk, disorder, and adaptation*. New York: Wiley.

Dolan, L. J., Kellam, S. G., Brown, C. H., Werthamer-Larsson, L., Rebok, G. W., Mayer, L. S., Laudolff, J., Turkkan, J. S., Ford, C., & Wheeler, L. (1993). The short-term impact of two classroom-based preventive interventions on aggressive and shy behaviors and poor achievement. *Journal of Applied Developmental Psychology, 14*(3), 317–345.

Drummond, T. (1993). *The Student Risk Screening Scale (SRSS)*. Grants Pass, OR: Josephine County Mental Health Program.

Dumas, J. E., Blechman, E. A., & Prinz, R. J. (1994). Aggressive children and effective communication. *Aggressive Behavior, 20*, 347–358.

Dwyer, K., Osher, D., & Warger, C. (1998). *Early warning: Timely response: A guide to safe schools*. Washington, DC: U.S. Department of Education. Available at *www.ed.gov/offices/ OSERS/OSEP/Products/ActionGuide/*

Eber, L., Nelson, C. M., & Miles, P. (1997). School-based wraparound for students with emotional and behavioral challenges. *Exceptional Children, 63*, 539–555.

Eddy, J. M., Reid, J. B., & Fetrow, R. A. (2000). An elementary school-based prevention program targeting modifiable antecedents of youth delinquency and violence. *Journal of Emotional and Behavioral Disorders, 8*, 165–176.

Egan, S. K., & Perry, D. G. (1998). Does low self-regard invite victimization? *Developmental Psychology, 34*, 299–309.

Eggert, L. L., Thompson, E. A., Herting, J. R., & Randell, B. P. (2001). Reconnecting youth to prevent drug abuse, school dropout, and suicidal behaviors among high-risk youth. In E. Wagner & H. B. Waldron (Eds.), *Innovations in adolescent substance abuse intervention*. Oxford, UK: Elsevier Science.

Eggert, L.L., Thompson, E.A., Pike, K.C., & Randell, B.P. (2002). Preliminary effects of two brief school-based prevention approaches for reducing youth suicide-risk behaviors, depression, and drug involvement. *Journal of Child and Adolescent Psychiatric Nursing, 15*(2), 48–64.

Elias, M. J., Zins, J. E., Graczyk, P. A., & Weissberg, R. P. (2004). Implementation, sustainability, and scaling up of social–emotional and academic innovations in public schools. *School Psychology Review, 32*(3), 303–319.

Embry, D. D. (2004). Community-based prevention using simple, low-cost, evidence-based kernels and behavior vaccines. *Journal of Community Psychology, 32*, 1–17.

Embry, D. D., & Flannery, D. J. (1994). *Peacebuilders—reducing youth violence: A working application of cognitive–social–imitative competence research*. Tucson, AZ: Heartsprings.

Epstein, J. (1992). School and family partnerships. In M. C. Alkin (Ed.), *Encyclopedia of educational research* (6th ed.). New York: Macmillan.

Epstein, M. H., & Sharma, J. (1998). *Behavioral and emotional rating scale*. Austin, TX: PRO-ED.

Epstein, M. H., & Walker, H. M. (2002). Special education: Best practices and First Step to Success. In B. J. Burns & K. Hoagwood (Eds.), *Community treatment for youth: Evidence-based interventions for severe emotional and behavioral disorders*. New York: Oxford University Press.

Espelage, D. L., Bosworth, K., & Simon, T. R. (2001). Short-term stability and prospective correlates of bullying in middle-school students: An examination of potential demographic, psychological, and environmental influences. *Violence and Victims, 16,* 411–426.

Espelage, D. L., & Swearer, S. (2003). Mini-series: Bullying prevention and intervention: Integrating research and evaluation findings: Research on school bullying and victimization: What have we learned and where do we go from here? *School Psychology Review, 32*(3), 365–384.

Evelo, D., Sinclair, M., Hurley, C., Christenson, S., & Thurlow, M. (1996). *Keeping kids in school: Using check and connect for dropout prevention.* Minneapolis: University of Minnesota Press.

Fashola, O. S., & Slavin, R. E. (1997). *Effective and replicable programs for students placed at risk in elementary and middle schools.* Washington DC: U.S. Department of Education, Office of Educational Research and Improvement. Available at *http://www.successforall.com/resource/research/effective.htm*

Feil, E., Severson, H., & Walker, H. (1994). *Early screening project: Identifying preschool children with adjustment problems* (Oregon Conference Monograph, Vol. 6). Eugene: University of Oregon.

Feil, E., Severson, H., & Walker, H. (2002). Early screening and intervention to prevent the development of aggressive, destructive behavior patterns among at-risk children. In M. Shinn, H. Walker, & G. Stoner (Eds.), *Interventions for academic and behavior problems II: Preventive and remedial approaches.* Bethesda, MD: National Association of School Psychologists.

Fein, R. A., Vossekuil, B., Pollack, W., Borum, R., Modzeleski, W., & Reddy, M. (2002). *Threat assessment in schools: A guide to managing threatening situations and creating safe school climates.* Washington, DC: Department of Education, U.S. Secret Service.

Franca, V. M., Kerr, M. M., Reitz, A. L., & Lambert, D. (1990). Peer tutoring among behaviorally disordered students: Academic and social benefits to tutor and tutee. *Education and Treatment of Children, 13,* 109–128.

Frazier, P. (1990). Victims' attributions and post-rape trauma. *Journal of Personality and Social Psychology, 59,* 298–304.

Frey, K. S., Hirschstein, M. K., & Guzzo, B. A. (2000). Second step: Preventing aggression by promoting social competence. In M. Epstein & H. Walker (Eds.), *Making schools safer and violence free: Critical issues, solutions, and recommended practices.* Austin, TX: PRO-ED.

Frey, L. M. (2003). Abundant beautification: An effective service-learning project for students with emotional or behavioral disorders. *Teaching Exceptional Children, 35,* 66–75.

Furlong, M. J., & Morrison, G. M. (Eds.). (1994). School violence and safety in perspective (9-article miniseries). *School Psychology Review, 23*(2), 139–261.

Furlong, M. J., & Morrison, R. L. (2000). The school in school violence: Definitions and facts. In H. Walker & M. Epstein (Eds.), *Making schools safer and violence free: Critical issues, solutions, and recommended practices.* Austin, TX: PRO-ED.

Galen, B. R., & Underwood, M. K. (1997). A developmental investigation of social aggression among children. *Developmental Psychology, 33,* 589–600.

Garrity, C., Jens, K., Porter, W., Sager, N., & Short-Camilli, C. (1994). *Bully-proofing your school.* Longmont, CO: Sopris West.

Ge, X., Conger, R. D., Lorenz, R. O., & Simons, R. L. (1994). Parents' stressful life events and adolescent depressed mood. *Journal of Health and Social Behavior, 35,* 28–44.

Gerber, M. M., & Semmel, M. I. (1984). Teacher as imperfect test: Reconceptualizing the referral process. *Educational Psychologist, 19*(3), 137–148.

Goldstein, A. P. (1999). Aggression reduction strategies: Effective and ineffective. *School Psychology Quarterly, 14,* 40–58.

Golly, A., Sprague, J., Walker, H. M., Beard, K., & Gorham, G. (2000). The First Step to Success program: An analysis of outcomes with identical twins across multiple baselines. *Behavioral Disorders, 25,* 170–182.

Gottfredson, D. C. (1987). Developing effective organizations to reduce school disorder. In O. C. Moles (Ed.), *Strategies to reduce student misbehavior.* Washington, DC: Office of Educational Research and Improvement.

Gottfredson, D. C. (1997). School-based crime prevention. In L. Sherman, D. Gottfredson, D. Mackenzie, J. Eck, P. Reuter, & S. Bushway (Eds.), *Preventing crime: What works, what doesn't, what's promising.* College Park, MD: Department of Criminology and Criminal Justice, University of Maryland.

Gottfredson, D. C. (2001). *Schools and delinquency.* New York: Cambridge University Press.

Gottfredson, D. C., Gottfredson, G. D., & Hybl, L. G. (1993). Managing adolescent behavior: A multiyear, multischool study. *American Educational Research Journal, 30,* 179–215.

Gottfredson, G. D. (1984). *The Effective School Battery.* Odessa, FL: Psychological Assessment Resources Incorporated.

Gottfredson, G. D., & Gottfredson, D. C. (1985). *Victimization in schools.* New York: Plenum Press.

Gottfredson, G. D., Gottfredson, D. C., & Czeh, E. R. (2000). *National study of delinquency prevention in schools* (Final Report, Grant No. 96-MU-MU-0008). Ellicott City, MD: Gottfredson Associates, Inc.

Graham, S., & Juvonen, J. (2001). An attributional approach to peer victimization. In J. Juvonen & S. Graham (Eds.), *Peer harassment in school.* New York: Guilford Press.

Green, M. (1999). *The appropriate and effective use of security technologies in U.S. schools: A guide for schools and law enforcement agencies* (Sandia National Laboratories, National Institute of Justice Research Report). Washington, DC: U.S. Department of Justice.

Greenberg, M. T., Domitrovich, C., & Bumbarger, B. (1999). *Preventing mental disorders in school-age children: A review of the effectiveness of prevention programs* (report submitted to Center for Mental Health Services, Substance Abuse Mental Health Services Administration). Washington, DC: U.S. Department of Health and Human Services.

Greenwood, C., Walker, H. M., Todd, N., & Hops, H. (1979). Selecting a cost-effective device for the assessment of social withdrawal. *Journal of Applied Behavior Analysis, 12,* 639–652.

Gresham, F. M., & Elliott, S. (1990). *Social Skills Rating System.* Circle Pines, MN: American Guidance Service.

Gresham, F. M., Lane, K. L., MacMillan, D. L., & Bocian, K. M. (1999). Social and academic profiles of externalizing and internalizing groups: Risk factors for emotional and behavioral disorders. *Behavioral Disorders, 24*(3), 231–245.

Grossman, D. C., Neckerman, H. J., Koepsell, T. D., Liu, P. Y., Asher, K. N., Beland, K., Frey, K., & Rivara, F. P. (1997). Effectiveness of a violence prevention curriculum among children in elementary school: A randomized controlled trial. *Journal of the American Medical Association, 277*(20), 1605–1611.

Grossman, J. B., & Garry, E. M. (1997). *Mentoring: A proven delinquency prevention strategy.* Washington, DC: Office of Juvenile Justice and Delinquency Programs, U.S. Department of Justice.

Hallinger, P., & Heck, R. H. (1998). Exploring the principal's contribution to school effectiveness: 1980–1995. *School Effectiveness and School Improvement, 9*(2), 157–191.

Harrington, R., Rutter, M., & Fombonne, E. (1996). Developmental pathways in depression: Multiple meanings, antecedents, and end-points. *Development and Psychopathology, 8,* 601–616.

Hawkins, D., & Catalano, R. (1992). *Communities that care.* San Francisco: Jossey-Bass.

Hawkins, J. D., Catalano, R. F., Kosterman, R., Abbott, R., & Hill, K. G. (1999). Preventing adolescent health-risk behaviors by strengthening protection during childhood. *Archives of Pediatrics and Adolescent Medicine, 153,* 226–234.

Hawkins, J. D., Catalano, R. F., Morrison, D., O'Donnell, J., Abbott, R., & Day, E. (1992). The Seattle Social Development Project: Effects of the first four years on protective factors and problem behaviors. In J. McCord & R. E. Tremblay (Eds.), *Preventing antisocial behavior: Interventions from birth through adolescence.* New York: Guilford Press.

Hawkins, J. D., Von Cleve, E., & Catalano, R. F. (1991). Reducing early childhood aggression: Results of a primary prevention program. *Journal of the American Academy of Child and Adolescent Psychiatry, 30,* 208–217.

Henderson, A., & Berla, N. (Eds.). (1994). *A new generation of evidence: The family is critical to student achievement.* Washington, DC: National Committee for Citizens in Education, Center for Law and Education.

Henggeler, S. W., Edwards, J., & Borduin, C. M. (1987). The family relations of female juvenile delinquents. *Journal of Abnormal Child Psychology, 15,* 199–209.

Henggeler, S. W., Mihalic, S. F., Rone, L., Thomas, C., & Timmons-Mitchell, J. (1998). *Blueprints for violence prevention, Book 6: Multisystemic therapy.* Boulder, CO: Center for the Study and Prevention of Violence.

Henry, D., Guerra, N., Huesmann, R., Tolan, P., Van Acker, R., & Erin, L. (2000). Normative influences on aggression in urban elementary school classrooms. *American Journal of Community Psychology, 28,* 59–81.

Herrera, C. (1999). *School-based mentoring: A first look into its potential.* Philadelphia: Public/Private Ventures.

Herrera, C., Sipe, C. L., & McClanahan, W. S. (2000). Mentoring school-age children: Relationship development in community-based and school-based programs.

Hodges, E. V., Finnegan, R. A., & Perry, D. (1999). Skewed autonomy-relatedness in preadolescents' conceptions of their relationships with mother, father and best friend. *Developmental Psychology, 35,* 737–748.

Hoover, J. H., Oliver, R., & Hagler, R. J. (1992). Bullying: Perceptions of adolescent victims in the Midwestern U.S.A. *School Psychology International, 13,* 5–16.

Horner, R. H., Sugai, G., Lewis-Palmer, T., & Todd, A. (2001). Teaching school-wide behavioral expectations. *Report on Emotional and Behavioral Disorders in Youth, 1*(4), 77–80.

Horner, R. H., Todd, A. W., Lewis-Palmer, T., Irvin, L. K., Sugai, G., & Boland, J. B. (2004). The School-Wide Evaluation Tool (SET): A research instrument for assessing school-wide positive behavior support. *Journal of Positive Behavior Interventions,6*(1), 3–12.

Hudley, C., & Graham, S. (1992). An attributional intervention to reduce peer-directed aggression among African-American boys. *Child Development, 63,* 124–138.

Huesmann, L. R., & Guerra, N. (1997). Children's normative beliefs about aggression and aggressive behavior. *Journal of Personality and Social Psychology, 72,* 408–419.

Hughes, J., & Hasbrouck, J. (1996). Television violence: Implications for violence prevention. *School Psychology Review, 25*(2), 134–151.

Ingersoll, R. M. (2001). Teacher turnover and teacher shortages: An organizational analysis. *American Educational Research Journal, 38*(3), 499–534.

Irvin, L. K., Tobin, T. J., Sprague, J. R., Sugai, G., & Vincent, C. G. (2004). Validity of office discipline referrals measures as indices of school-wide behavioral status and effects of school-wide behavioral interventions. *Journal of Positive Behavior Interventions, 6*(31), 131–147.

Irvine, A. B., Biglan, A., Smolkowski, K., Metzler, C. W., & Ary, D. V. (1999). The effectiveness of a parenting skills program for parents of middle school students in small communities. *Journal of Consulting and Clinical Psychology, 67,* 811–825.

Jacobson, J., & Willie, D. (1986). The influence of attachment patterns on developmental changes in peer interaction from the toddler to the preschool period. *Child Development, 57,* 338–347.

Janoff-Bulman, R. (1979). Characterological and behavioral self-blame: Inquiries into depression and rape. *Journal of Personality and Social Psychology, 37,* 1798–1809.

Juvonen, J., & Graham, E. (2001). *Peer harassment in school: The plight of the vulnerable and victimized.* New York: Guilford Press.

Kacir, C., & Gordon, D. A. (1997). Interactive videodisk parent training for parents of difficult pre-teens. *Child and Family Behavior Therapy, 21*(4), 1–22.

Kam, C. M., Greenberg, M. T., & Walls, C. T. (2003). Examining the role of implementation quality in school-based prevention using the PATHS curriculum. *Prevention Science, 4*(1), 55–63.

Kamps, D., Kravits, T., Rauch, J., Kamps, J. L., & Chung, N. (2000). A prevention program for students with or at risk for ED: Moderating effects of variation in treatment and classroom structure. *Journal of Emotional and Behavioral Disorders, 8,* 141–154.

Katz, M. (1997). *On playing a poor hand well: Insights from the lives of those who have overcome childhood risks and adversities.* New York: Norton.

Kauffman, J. (1999). *Early identification of emotionally handicapped children in school.* Springfield, IL: Thomas.

Kauffman, J. (2003). Appearances, stigma, and prevention. *Remedial and Special Education, 24,* 195–198.

Kauffman, J. (2004). How we prevent the prevention of emotional and behavioral difficulties in education. In P. Garneer, F. Yuen, P. Clough, & T. Pardeck (Eds.), *Handbook of emotional and behavioral difficulties in education.* London: Sage.

Kaufman, P., Chen, X., Choy, S. P., Ruddy, S. A., Miller, A. K., Fleury, J. K., Chandler, K. A., Rand, M. R., Klaus, P., & Planty, M. G. (2000). *Indicators of school crime and safety, 2000.* U.S. Department of Education (NCES 2001-017) and U.S. Department of Justice (NCJ-184176). Washington, DC. Available at: *nces.ed.gov/pubs2001/quarterly/winter/elementary/e_section4.html*

Kazdin, A. (1993). Treatment of conduct disorder: Progress and directions in psychotherapy research. *Development and Psychotherapy, 5*(1/2), 277–310.

Kazdin, A. E. (1997). Parent management training: Evidence, outcomes, and issues. *Journal of the American Academy of Child and Adolescent Psychiatry, 36,* 1249–1357.

Kearney, C. A., & Tillotson, C. A. (1998). School attendance. In T. S. Watson & F. M. Grsham (Eds.), *Handbook of child behavior therapy.* New York: Plenum Press.

Kellam, S. G., Ling, X., Merisca, R., Brown, C. H., & Ialongo, N. (1998). The effect of the level of aggression in the first grade classroom on the course and malleability of aggressive behavior into middle school. *Development and Psychopathology, 10,* 165–185.

Kellam, S. G., Mayer, L. S., Rebok, G. W., & Hawkins, W. E. (1998). The effects of improving achievement on aggressive behavior and of improving aggressive behavior on achievement through two preventive interventions: An investigation of causal paths. In B. P. Dohrenwend (Ed.), *Adversity, stress, and psychopathology.* New York: Oxford University Press.

Kellam, S., & Rebok, G.W. (1992). Building developmental and etiological theory through epidemiologically based preventive intervention trials. In J. McCord & R.E. Tremblay (Eds.), *Preventing antisocial behavior: Interventions from birth through adolescence.* New York: Guilford Press.

Kern, L., Dunlap, G., Clarke, S., & Childs, K. E. (1994). Student-assisted functional assessment interview. *Diagnostique, 19,* 29–39.

Kingery, P. (1999). Suspensions and expulsions: New directions. In *Effective violence prevention programs.* (Hamilton–Fish National Institute on School and Community Violence). Washington, DC: George Washington University.

Kingery, P. M., & Walker, H. M. (2002). What we know about school safety. In M. Shinn, H. Walker, & G. Stoner (Eds.), *Interventions for academic and behavior problems II: Preventive and remedial approaches.* Bethesda, MD: National Association of School Psychologists.

Knoff, H. M., & Batsche, G. M. (1995). Project ACHIEVE: Analyzing a school reform process for at-risk and underachieving students. *School Psychology Review, 24,* 579–603.

Kochenderfer, B., & Ladd, G. (1996). Peer victimization: Manifestations and relations to school adjustment in kindergarten. *Journal of School Psychology, 34,* 267–283.

Kochenderfer, B., & Ladd, G. (1997). Victimized children's responses to peer aggression: Behaviors associated with reduced versus continued victimization. *Development and Psychopathology, 9,* 59–73.

Kupersmidt, J., Patterson, C., & Eickholt, C. (1989). *Socially rejected children: Bullies, victims, or both? Aggressors, victims, and peer relationships.* Paper presented at the Society for Research in Child Development, Kansas City, MO.

Lane, K. (2003). Identifying young students at risk for antisocial behavior: The utility of "Teachers as Tests." *Behavioral Disorders, 28*(4), 360–369.

Lareau, A. (1987). Social class differences in family–school relationships: The importance of cultural capital. *Sociology of Education, 60,* 288–301.

Leadbeater, B. J., Kuperminc, G. P., Blatt, S. J., & Hertzog, C. (1999). A multivariate model of gender differences in adolescents' internalizing and externalizing problems. *Developmental Psychology, 35,* 1268–1282.

LeBlanc, M. (1998). Screening of serious and violent juvenile offenders. In R. Loeber & D. Farrington (Eds.), *Serious and violent juvenile offenders.* Thousand Oaks, CA: Sage.

Leff, S. S., Power, T. J., Costigan, T. E., & Manz, P. H. (2003). Mini-series: Bullying prevention and intervention: Integrating research and evaluation findings. Assessing the climate of the playground and lunchroom: Implications for bullying prevention programming. *School Psychology Review, 32*(3), 418–431.

Levin, D. U., & Ornstein, A. (1989). Research on classroom and school effectiveness and its implications for improving big city schools. *Urban Review, 21,* 81–94.

Lewis, T. J., Sugai, G., & Colvin, G. (1998). Reducing problem behavior through a school-wide system of effective behavioral support: Investigation of a school-wide social skills training program and contextual interventions. *School Psychology Review, 27,* 446–459.

Lieberman, C. (1994, May). *Television and violence.* Paper presented at the Council of State Governments Conference on School Violence, Westlake Village, CA.

Limber, S. P., & Small, M. S. (2003). Mini-series: Bullying prevention and intervention: Integrating research and evaluation findings. State laws and policies to address bullying in schools. *School Psychology Review, 32*(3), 445–456.

Lipsey, M. W. (1991). The effect of treatment on juvenile delinquents: Results from meta-analysis. In F. Losel, D. Bender, & T. Bliesener (Eds.), *Psychology and law.* New York: de Gruyter.

Lloyd, J. W., Forness, S. R., & Kavale, K. A. (1998). Some methods are more effective than others. *Intervention in School and Clinic, 33,* 195–200.

Lloyd, J. W., Kauffman, J. M., Landrum, T. J., & Roe, D. L. (1991). Why do teachers refer pupils for special education?: An analysis of referral records. *Exceptionality, 2*(3), 115–126.

Lochman, J. E., Burch, P. R., Curry, J. F., & Lampron, L. B. (1984). Treatment and generalization effects of cognitive-behavioral and goal-setting interventions with aggressive boys. *Journal of Consulting and Clinical Psychology, 52,* 915–916.

Lochman, J. E., Coie, J. D., Underwood, M. K., & Terry, R. (1993). Effectiveness of a social relations intervention program for aggressive and nonaggressive rejected children. *Journal of Consulting and Clinical Psychology, 61*(6), 1053–1058.

Loeber, R., Dishion, T. J., & Patterson, G. R. (1984). Multiple gating: A multi-stage assessment procedure for identifying youths at risk for delinquency. *Journal of Research in Crime and Delinquency, 21*(1), 7–32.

Loeber, R., & Farrington, D. P. (1998a). Never too early, never too late: Risk factors and successful intervention for serious and violent juvenile offenders. *Studies on Crime and Crime Prevention, 7*(1), 7–30.

Loeber, R., & Farrington, D. (Eds.). (1998b). *Serious and violent juvenile offenders: Risk factors and successful interventions.* Thousand Oaks, CA: Sage.

Loeber, R., & Farrington, D. (Eds.). (2001). *Child delinquents: Development, intervention and service needs.* Thousand Oaks, CA: Sage.

Loeber, R., Green, S. M., Keenan, K., & Lahey, B. B. (1995). Which boys will fare worse?: Early predictors of the onset of conduct disorder in a six-year longitudinal study. *Journal of the American Academy of Child and Adolescent Psychiatry, 34,* 499–509.

Loeber, R., & Hay, D. (1997). Key issues in the development of aggression and violence from childhood to early adulthood. *Annual Review of Psychology, 48,* 371–410.

Martens, B. K., & Kelly, S. Q. (1993). A behavioral analysis of effective teaching. *School Psychology Quarterly, 8,* 10–26.

Mathur, S. R., Kavale, K. A., Quinn, M. M., Forness, S. R., & Rutherford, R. B. (1998). Social skills interventions with students with emotional and behavioral problems: A quantitative synthesis of single-subject research. *Behavioral Disorders, 23,* 193–201.

May, S., Ard, B., Todd, A., Horner, R., Glasgow, A., Sugai, G., & Sprague, J. R. (2001). *SWIS user's manual: Learning to use the school-wide information system.* Eugene: Center on Positive Behavioral Interventions and Supports, University of Oregon.

Mayer, G. R. (1995). Preventing antisocial behavior in the schools. *Journal of Applied Behavioral Analysis, 28,* 467–478.

McEvoy, A., & Welker, R. (2000). Antisocial behavior, academic failure, and school climate: A critical review. In H. Walker & M. Epstein (Eds.), *Making schools safer and violence free: Critical issues, solutions, and recommended practices.* Austin, TX: PRO-ED.

McPartland, J. A., & Nettles, S. M. (1991). Using community adults as advocates or mentors for at-risk middle school students: A two-year evaluation of Project RAISE. *American Journal of Education, 99,* 568–586.

Merrell, K. W. (1993). Using behavior rating scales to assess social skills and antisocial behavior in school settings: Development of the school social behavior scales. *School Psychology Review, 22*(1), 115–133.

Merrell, K. W. (2001). Assessment of children's social skills: Recent developments, best practices, and new directions. *Exceptionality, 9*(1 & 2), 3–18.

Merrell, K. W. (2002a). *Preschool and kindergarten behavior scales* (2nd ed.). Austin, TX: PRO-ED.

Merrell, K. W. (2002b). *School social behavior scales* (2nd ed.). Eugene, OR: Assessment-Intervention Resources (*http://www.assessment-intervention.com*).

Merrell, K. W. (2003). *Behavioral, social, and emotional assessment of children and adolescents* (2nd ed.). Mahwah, NJ: Erlbaum.

Messick, S. (1988). The once and future issues of validity: Assessing the meaning and consequences of measurement. In H. Wainer & H. Braun (Eds.), *Test validity.* Hillsdale, NJ: Erlbaum.

Metzler, C. W., Biglan, A., Rusby, J. C., & Sprague, J. R. (2001). Evaluation of a comprehensive behavior management program to improve school-wide positive behavior support. *Education and Treatment of Children, 24*(4), 448–479.

Miedel, W. T., & Reynolds, A. J. (1999). Parent involvement in early intervention for disadvantaged children: Does it matter? *Journal of School Psychology, 37,* 379–399.

Mihalic, S., Irwin, K., Elliott, D., Fagan, A., & Hansen, D. (2001). *Blueprints for violence prevention, Juvenile Justice Bulletin.* Washington DC: Office of Juvenile Justice and Delinquency Prevention, U.S. Department of Justice.

Nansel, T. R., Overpeck, M., Haynie, D. L., Ruan, J., & Scheidt, P. C. (2003). Relationships between bullying and violence among U.S. youth. *Archives of Pediatrics and Adolescent Medicine, 157*(4), 348–355.

Nansel, T. R., Overpeck, M., Pilla, R. S., Ruan, W. J., Simons-Morton, F., & Scheidt, P. (2001). Bullying behaviors among U.S. youth: Prevalence and association with psycho–social adjustment. *Journal of the American Medical Association, 285*(16), 2094–2100.

Nelson, J. R. (2000). Designing schools to meet the needs of students who exhibit disruptive behavior. In H. Walker & M. Epstein (Eds.), *Making schools safer and violence free: Critical issues, solutions, and recommended practices.* Austin, TX: PRO-ED.

Nelson, J. R., & Roberts, M. L. (2000). Ongoing reciprocal teacher–student interactions involving disruptive behaviors in general education classrooms. *Journal of Emotional and Behavioral Disorders, 8,* 27–37.

Nelson, J. R., Smith, D. J., Young, R. K., & Dodd, J. M. (1991). A review of self-management outcome research conducted with students who exhibit behavioral disorders. *Behavioral Disorders, 16,* 169–179.

Newton, F. R. (1994). A study of the effectiveness of using collegiate mentors to reduce violent behavior, improve self-concept, and increase academic success in an urban middle school (at risk). *Dissertation Abstracts International, 55*(06-A), 1440. (UMI No. AAD94-29678)

O'Donnell, J., Hawkins, J., Catalano, R., Abbott, R., & Day, L. (1995). Preventing school failure, drug use, and delinquency among low-income children: Long-term intervention in elementary schools. *American Journal of Orthopsychiatry, 65,* 87–100.

Office of Juvenile Justice and Delinquency Prevention. (1993). *Weeklong OJJDP workshop on adolescent drug prevention.* San Jose, CA.

Olweus, D. (1978). *Aggression in the schools: Bullies and whipping boys.* Washington, DC: Hemisphere Press.

Olweus, D. (1991). Bully/victim problems among school children: Basic facts and effects of a school-based intervention program. In D. Pepler & K. Rubin (Eds.), *The development and treatment of childhood aggression.* Hillsdale, NJ: Erlbaum.

Olweus, D. (1992). *The Olweus Bully/Victim Questionnaire.* Unpublished material. Research Center for Health Promotion (HEMIL), Christies gate 13, N-5015, Bergen, Norway.

Olweus, D. (1993). *Bullying at school.* Cambridge, MA: Blackwell.

Olweus, D. (1994). Bullying at school: Basic facts and effects of a school-based intervention program. *Journal of Child Psychology and Psychiatry, 35*(7), 1171–1190.

Olweus, D. (1996). Bullying at school: Knowledge base and an effective intervention program. *Annals of the New York Academy of Sciences, 794,* 265.

Olweus, D. (2001). Peer harassment: A critical analysis and some important issues. In J. Juvonen & S. Graham (Eds.), *Peer harassment in school: The plight of the vulnerable and victimized.* New York: Guilford Press.

Olweus, D., Limber, S., & Mihalic, S. (2000). *Blueprints for violence prevention, Book Nine: Bullying prevention program.* (Blueprints for Violence Prevention Series). Boulder, CO: Center for the Study and Prevention of Violence, University of Colorado.

O'Neill, R. E., Horner, R. H., Albin, R. W., Sprague, J. R., Newton, S., & Storey, K. (1997). *Functional assessment and program development for problem behavior: A practical handbook* (2nd ed.). Pacific Grove, CA: Brooks/Cole.

Orpinas, P., Horne, A. M., & Staniszewski, D. (2003). Mini-series: Bullying prevention and intervention: Integrating research and evaluation findings. School bullying: Changing the problem by changing the school. *School Psychology Review, 32*(3), 431–445.

Osher, D., Dwyer, K., & Jackson, S. (2003). *Safe, supportive and successful schools: Step by step.* Longmont, CO: Sopris West.

O'Toole, M. E. (2000). *The school shooter: A threat assessment perspective.* Quantico, VA: Critical Incident Response Group (CIRG), National Center for the Analysis of Violent Crime (NCAVC), FBI Academy, Federal Bureau of Investigation.

Paine, C. (2002). Preparing for and managing school crises. In M. Shinn, H. Walker, & G. Stoner (Eds.), *Interventions for academic and behavior problems II: Preventive and remedial approaches.* Bethesda, MD: National Association of School Psychologists.

Paine, C. K., & Sprague, J. (2002). Dealing with a school shooting disaster: Lessons learned from Springfield, Oregon. *Emotional and Behavioral Disorders in Youth, 2*(2), 35–40.

Patterson, G. R., Reid, J. B., & Dishion, T. J. (1992). *Antisocial boys. Vol. 4. A social interactional approach.* Eugene, OR: Castalia Press.

Pellegrini, A. D. (2001). Rough and tumble play from childhood through adolescence: Development and possible functions. In P. K. Smith & C. H. Hart (Eds.), *Childhood social development.* Malden, MA: Blackwell.

Pellegrini, A. D., & Bartini, M. (2000). An empirical comparison of sampling aggression and victimization in school settings. *Journal of Educational Psychology, 92,* 360–366.

Perry, D., Hodges, E., & Egan, S. (2001). Determinants of chronic victimization by peers: A review and new model of family influence. In J. Juvonen & S. Graham (Eds.), *Peer harassment in school: The plight of the vulnerable and victimized.* New York: Guilford Press.

Perry, D., Kusel, S. J., & Perry, L.C. (1988). Victims of peer aggression. *Developmental Psychology, 24,* 807–814.

Perry, D., Perry, L., & Kennedy, E. (1992). Conflict and the development of antisocial behavior. In C. U. Shantz & W. Hartup (Eds.), *Conflict in child and adolescent development.* New York: Cambridge University Press.

Peterson, K. D., Bennet, B., & Sherman, D. F. (1991). Themes of uncommonly successful teachers of at-risk students. *Urban Education, 26,* 176–194.

Plake, B. S., Impara, J. C., & Spies, A. (2003). *The fifteenth mental measurements yearbook.* Omaha: University of Nebraska Press.

Poole, C. (1997). Up with emotional health. *Educational Leadership, 54,* 12–14.

Ramsey, E., & Walker, H. M. (1988). Family management correlates of antisocial behavior among middle school boys. *Behavioral Disorders, 13,* 187–201.

Raywid, M. A. (1990). Alternative education: The definition problem. *Changing Schools, 18,* 4–5.

Redden, S., Forness, S., Ramey, S., Ramey, C., Zima, B., Brezausek, C., & Kavale, K. (1999). Head Start children at third grade: Preliminary special education identification and placement of children with emotional, learning, and related disabilities. *Journal of Child and Family Studies, 8*(3), 285–303.

Reed, H., Thomas, E., Sprague, J. R., & Horner, R. H. (1997). The student guided functional assessment interview: An analysis of student and teacher agreement. *Journal of Behavioral Education, 7,* 33–49.

Reid, J. B. (1991). Mediational screening as a model for prevention research. *American Journal of Community Psychology, 19,* 867–872.

Reid, J. B. (1993). Prevention of conduct disorder before and after school entry: Relating interventions to developmental findings. *Development and Psychopathology, 5*(1/2), 243–262.

Reid, J. B., Eddy, J. M., Fetrow, R. A., & Stoolmiller, M. (1999). Description and immediate impacts of a preventive intervention for conduct problems. *American Journal of Community Psychology, 27,* 483–517.

Reid, J. B., Patterson, G. R., & Snyder, J. (Eds.). (2002). *Antisocial behavior in children and adolescents: A developmental analysis and the Oregon Model for Intervention.* Washington, DC: American Psychological Association.

Resnick, M. D., Bearman, P. S., Blum, R. W., Bauman, K. E., Harris, K. M., Jones, J., Tabor, T., Beuhring, T., Sieving, R. E., Shew, M., Ireland, M., Tearinger, L. H., & Udry, J. R. (1997). Protecting adolescents from harm: Findings from the National Longitudinal Study on Adolescent Health. *Journal of the American Medical Association, 278,* 823–836.

Rigby, K. (2001). Health consequences of bullying and its prevention in schools. In J. Juvonen & S. Graham (Eds.), *Peer harassment in school: The plight of the vulnerable and victimized.* New York: Guilford Press.

Rodkin, P. C., & Hodges, E. V. (2003). Bullies and victims in the peer ecology: Four questions for psychologists and school professionals. *School Psychology Review, 32*(3), 384–400.

Romer, D., & Heller, T. (1983). Social adaptation of mentally retarded adults in community settings: A social–ecological approach. *Applied Research in Mental Retardation, 4,* 303–314.

Rosenthal, S. L., & Simeonsson, R. L. (1991). Communication skills in emotionally disturbed and nondisturbed adolescents. *Behavioral Disorders, 16,* 192–199.

Ross, A. (1980). *Psychological disorders of children: A behavioral approach to theory, research and therapy* (2nd ed.). New York: McGraw-Hill.

Salmivalli, C. (2001). Group view on victimization: Empirical findings and their implications. In J. Juvonen & S. Graham (Eds.), *Peer harassment in school: The plight of the vulnerable and victimized.* New York: Guilford Press.

Satcher, D. (2001). *Youth violence: A report of the Surgeon General.* Washington, DC: U.S. Department of Health and Human Services.

Schneider, T., Walker, H. M., & Sprague, J. R. (2001). *Safe school design: A handbook for educational leaders.* Eugene: ERIC Clearinghouse on Educational Management, College of Education, University of Oregon.

Schwartz, D., Proctor, L. J., & Chen, D. H. (2001). The aggressive victim of bullying: Emotional and behavioral dysregulation as a pathway to victimization by peers. In J. Juvonen & S. Graham (Eds.), *Peer harassment in school: The plight of the vulnerable and victimized.* New York: Guilford Press.

Schweinhart, L. J., Barnes, H. V., & Weikart, D. P. (1993). Significant benefits: The High/Scope Perry Preschool Study through age 27. *Monographs of the High/Scope Educational Research Foundation* (No. 10). Ypsilanti, MI: High/Scope Press.

Seale, A. (2002). The aftermath of bullying. *The Bulletin: The Newsletter of the Hamilton Fish Institute, 1*(2), 2. Washington, DC: George Washington University.

Segal, D., Chen, P.Y., Kacir, C.Y., & Gyglys, J. (2003). Development and evaluation of a parenting intervention program: Integration of scientific and practical approaches. *International Journal of Human–Computer Interaction, 15,* 453–468.

Shaw, D. S., Winslow, E. B., Owens, E. B., & Hood, N. (1998). Young children's adjustment to chronic family adversity: A longitudinal study of low-income families. *Journal of the American Academy of Child and Adolescent Psychiatry, 37,* 545–553.

Shield, A. M., Cicchetti, D., & Ryan, R. M. (1994). The development of emotional and behavioral self-regulation and social competence among maltreated school-age children. *Development and Psychopathology, 6,* 57–75.

Shure, M. B., & Spivac, G. (1980). Interpersonal problem-solving as a mediator of a behavioral adjustment in preschool and kindergarten children. *Journal of Applied Developmental Psychology, 1,* 29–44.

Simcha-Fagan, O., Langner, T., Gersten, J., & Eisenberg, J. (1975). *Violent and antisocial behavior: A longitudinal study of violent youth* (OCD-CB-480). Unpublished report of the Office of Child Development.

Sipe, C. (1996). *Mentoring: A synthesis of P/PV's reearch: 1988–1995.* Philadelphia: Public/Private Ventures.

Skiba, R., Peterson, R., & Williams, T. (1997). Office referrals and suspension: Disciplinary intervention in middle schools. *Education and Treatment of Children, 20*(3), 295–315.

Smith, C., & Carlson, B. E. (1997). Stress, coping, and resilience in children and youth. *Social Service Review, 71,* 231–247.

Smith, C. A., & Stern, S. B. (1997). Delinquency and antisocial behavior: A review of family processes and intervention research. *Social Service Review, 71,* 382–421.

Smith, S. G., & Sprague, J. R. (2001, March). *Rate and prevalence of bullying and harassment in a middle school: Results of a school-wide student, staff, and parent survey.* Paper presented at the Oregon Conference, Eugene, OR.

Smith, S. G., & Sprague, J. R. (2003). The mean kid: An overview of bully/victim problems and research-based solutions for schools. *Oregon School Study Council Bulletin, 44*(2).

Smith, S. G., Sprague, J. R., Myers, D., & Anderson, M. (2000, March). *Rate and prevalence of bullying and harassment in an elementary school: Results of a school-wide student, staff, and parent survey.* Paper presented at the Oregon Conference, Eugene, OR.

Snell, J. L., MacKenzie, E., & Frey, K. (2002). Bullying prevention in elementary schools: The importance of adult leadership, peer group support, and student social–emotional skills. In M. Shinn, H. Walker, & G. Stoner (Eds.), *Interventions for academic and behavior problems II: Preventive and remedial approaches.* Bethesda, MD: National Association of School Psychologists.

Soriano, M. (1994, Winter). The family's role in violence prevention and response. *School Safety,* 12–16.

Sprague, J. R., Colvin, G., & Irvin, L. K. (1995). *The Oregon School Safety Survey.* Eugene: University of Oregon.

Sprague, J. R., Colvin, G., Irvin, L. K., & Stieber, S. (1997a). *The Oregon School Safety Survey.* Available from the Institute on Violence and Destructive Behavior, 1265 University of Oregon, Eugene, OR 97403-1265.

Sprague, J. R., Colvin, G., Irvin, L. K., & Stieber, S. (1997b). *Assessing school safety in Oregon: How do school principals respond?* Available from the Institute on Violence and Destructive Behavior, 1265 University of Oregon, Eugene, OR 97403-1265.

Sprague, J. R., & Golly, A. (2004). *Best behavior: Building positive behavior supports in schools.* Longmont, CO: Sopris West.

Sprague, J.R., & Horner, R.H. (1999). Low frequency, high intensity problem behavior: Toward an applied technology of functional assessment and intervention. In A. C. Repp & R. H. Horner (Eds.), *Functional analysis of problem behavior: From effective assessment to effective support*. Pacific Grove, CA: Wadsworth.

Sprague, J. R., Sugai, G., Horner, R. H., & Walker, H. M. (1999). Using office discipline referral data to evaluate school-wide discipline and violence prevention interventions. *Oregon School Study Council Bulletin, 42*(2). Eugene: University of Oregon.

Sprague, J. R., Sugai, G., & Walker, H. (1998). Antisocial behavior in schools. In T. S. Watson & F. M. Gresham (Eds.), *Handbook of child behavior therapy*. New York: Plenum Press.

Sprague, J., & Walker, H. (2000). Early identification and intervention for youth with antisocial and violent behavior. *Exceptional Children, 66*(3), 367–379.

Sprague, J. R., Walker, H. M., Golly, A., White, K., Myers, D. R., & Shannon, T. (2001). Translating research into effective practice: The effects of a universal staff and student intervention on indicators of discipline and school safety. *Education and Treatment of Children, 24*(4), 495–511.

Sprague, J. R., Walker, H., Nishioka, V., Tobin, T., Bullis, M., & Eisert, D. C. (2001). *Skills for success: A violence prevention intervention for socially maladjusted middle school students*. University of Oregon, Institute on Violence and Destructive Behavior, Eugene, OR.

Sprague, J. R., Walker, H. M., Sowards, S., Bloem, C. V., Eberhardt, P., & Marshall, B. (2002). Sources of vulnerability to school violence: Systems-level assessment and strategies to improve safety and climate. In M. R. Shinn, H. M. Walker, & G. Stoner (Eds.), *Interventions for academic and behavior problems II: Preventive and remedial approaches*. Bethesda, MD: National Association of School Psychologists.

Sprague, J. R., Walker, H. M., Steiber, S., Simonsen, B., & Nishioka, V. (2001). Exploring the relationship between school discipline referrals and delinquency. *Psychology in the Schools, 38*, 197–206.

Stanger, C., Achenbach, T. M., & McConaughy, S. H. (1993). Three-year course of behavioral/emotional problems in a national sample of 4- to 16-year-olds: Predictors of signs of disturbance. *Journal of Consulting and Clinical Psychology, 61*, 839–848.

Stanley, P. D., Dai, Y., & Nolan, R. F. (1997). Differences in depression and self-esteem reported by learning disabled and behavior disordered middle school students. *Journal of Adolescence, 20*, 219–222.

Stephens, R. D. (1995). *Safe schools: A handbook for violence prevention*. Bloomington, IN: National Education Service.

Stevens, R. J., & Slavin, R. E. (1995). The cooperative elementary school: Effects on students' achievement, attitudes, and social relations. *American Educational Research Journal*, 321–351.

Stoiber, K. C., & Good, B. (1998). Risk and resilience factors linked to problem behavior among urban, culturally diverse adolescents. *School Psychology Review, 27*, 380–397.

Sugai, G., & Horner, R. (1994). Including students with severe behavior problems in general education settings: Assumptions, challenges, and solutions. *Oregon Conference Monograph, 6*, 102–120.

Sugai, G., & Horner, R. H. (2002). The evolution of discipline practices: School-wide positive behavior supports. *Child and Family Behavior Therapy, 24*, 23–50.

Sugai, G., Horner, R. H., & Gresham, F. (2002). Behaviorally effective environments. In M. R. Shinn, H. M. Walker, & G. Stoner (Eds.), *Interventions for academic and behavior problems II: Preventive and remedial approaches*. Bethesda, MD: National Association for School Psychologists.

Sugai, G., & Lewis, T. J. (Eds.). (1999). Developing positive behavioral support for students with challenging behaviors. *Miniseries Monograph of the International Conference for Children with Behavior Disorders*.

Sugai, G., Lewis-Palmer, T., & Hagan, S. (1998). Using functional assessments to develop behavior support plans. *Preventing School Failure, 43*, 6–13.

Sugai, G., Lewis-Palmer, T., Todd, A. W., & Horner, R. H. (1999). Systems-Wide Evaluation Tool: School Wide (SET-SW; Version 2.0). College of Education, University of Oregon, Eugene, OR.

Sugai, G., Lewis-Palmer, T., Todd, A., & Horner, R. (2000). *Effective Behavior Support (EBS) survey: Assessing and planning behavior support in schools*. Eugene: University of Oregon.

Sugai, G., Sprague, J. R., Horner, R. H., & Walker, H. M. (2000). Preventing school violence: The use of office discipline referrals to assess and monitor school-wide discipline interventions. *Journal of Emotional and Behavioral Disorders, 8*(2), 94–101.

Szapocznik, J., & Williams, R.A. (2000). Brief strategic family therapy: Twenty-five years of interplay among theory, research and practice in adolescent behavior problems and drug abuse. *Clinical Child and Family Psychology Review, 3*(2), 117–135.

Taylor-Greene, S., Brown, D., Nelson, L., Longton, J., Gassman, T., Cohen, J., Swartz, J., Horner, R. H., Sugai, G., & Hall, S. (1997). School-wide behavioral support: Starting the year off right. *Journal of Behavioral Education, 7*(1), 99–112.

Thompson, R. W., Ruma, P. R., Schuchmann, L. F., & Burks, R. V. (1995). A cost-effectiveness evaluation of parent training. *Journal of Child and Family Studies, 5*, 415–430.

Thornton, T. N., Craft, C. A., Dahlberg, L. L., Lynch, B. S., & Baer, K. (2000). *Best practices of youth violence prevention: A sourcebook for community action*. Atlanta: Centers for Disease Control and Prevention, National Center for Injury Prevention and Control.

Tiet, Q. Q., Bird, H. R., Davies, M., Hoven, C., Cohen, P., Jensen, P. S., & Goodman, S. (1998). Adverse life events and resilience. *Journal of the American Academy of Child and Adolescent Psychiatry, 37*, 1191–1201.

Tobin, T., & Sprague, J. (2000). Alternative education strategies: Reducing violence in school and community. *Journal of Emotional and Behavioral Disorders, 8*, 177–186.

Tobin, T., Sugai, G., & Colvin, G. (1996). Patterns in middle school discipline records. *Journal of Emotional and Behavioral Disorders, 4*(2), 82–94.

Tobin, T., Sugai, G., & Martin, E. (2000). *Final report for Project CREDENTIALS: Current research on educational endeavors to increase at-risk learners' success* (report submitted to the Office of Professional Technical Education, Oregon Department of Education). Eugene: College of Education, Behavioral Research and Teaching, University of Oregon.

Tolan, P. (1988). Socioeconomic, family, and social stress correlates of adolescent antisocial and delinquent behavior. *Journal of Abnormal Child Psychology, 16*, 317–331.

Tolan, P., Gorman-Smith, D., & Henry, D. (2001). New study to focus on efficacy of "whole school" prevention approaches. *Emotional and Behavioral Disorders in Youth.* 2(1), 5–7.

Tolan, P., & Guerra, N. (1994). *What works in reducing adolescent violence: An empirical review of the field.* Boulder: Center for the Study and Prevention of Violence, University of Colorado.

Troy, M., & Stroufe, L. A. (1987). Victimization among preschoolers: Role of attachment relationship history. *Journal of Child and Adolescent Psychiatry, 2,* 166–172.

Trump, K. (2000). *Classroom killers? Hallway hostages: How schools can prevent and manage school crises.* Thousand Oaks, CA: Corwin Press.

U.S. Department of Education. (1998). *National educational goals panel report.* Washington, DC: Author.

U.S. Department of Education Office for Civil Rights and the National Association of Attorneys General. (1999). *Protecting students from harassment and hate crime: A guide for schools.* Washington, DC: Author.

U.S. Department of Education Office of Safe and Drug-Free Schools. (2003). *Emergency planning for America's schools.* Retrieved December 19, 2003, from *www.ed.gov/admins/lead/safety/emergencyplan/index.html*

U.S. Departments of Justice and Education. (1998). *First annual report on school safety.* Washington, DC: Author.

U.S. Departments of Justice and Education. (1999). *Annual report on school safety.* Washington, DC: Author.

U.S. Departments of Justice and Education. (2000). *Annual report on school safety.* Washington, DC: Author.

Vance, J. E., Fernandez, B., & Biber, M. (1998). Educational progress in a population of youth with aggression and emotional disturbance: The role of risk and protective factors. *Journal of Emotional and Behavioral Disorders, 6,* 214–221.

Wahler, R., & Dumas, J. E. (1986). A chip off the old block: Some interpersonal characteristics of coercive children across generations. In P. Strain, M. Guralnick, & H. M. Walker (Eds.), *Children's social behavior: Development, assessment and modification.* Orlando, FL: Academic Press.

Walker, H. M. (1986). The Assessments for Integration into Mainstream Settings (AIMS) assessment system: Rationale, instruments, procedures, and outcomes. *Journal of Clinical Child Psychology, 15*(1), 55–63.

Walker, H. M. (1996). Violence prevention and school safety. In M. Quigley (Ed.), *Improving the implementation of the Individuals with Disabilities Act: Making schools work for all of America's children.* Washington, DC: National Council on Disability.

Walker, H. M. (1998). First steps to prevent antisocial behavior. *Teaching Exceptional Children, 30*(4), 16–19.

Walker, H. M., Block-Pedego, A., Todis, B., & Severson, H. (1991). *School archival records search (SARS): User's guide and technical manual.* Longmont, CO: Sopris West.

Walker, H. M., Colvin, G., & Ramsey, E. (1995). *Antisocial behavior in school: Strategies and best practices.* Pacific Grove, CA: Brooks/Cole.

Walker, H. M., & Eaton-Walker, J. (2000, March). Key questions about school safety: Critical issues and recommended solutions. *NASSP Bulletin (National Association of Secondary School Principals)*, 46–55.

Walker, H. M., Horner, R. H., Sugai, G., Bullis, M., Sprague, J. R., Bricker, D., & Kaufman, M. J. (1996). Integrated approaches to preventing antisocial behavior patterns among school-age children and youth. *Journal of Emotional and Behavioral Disorders, 4*(4), 194–209.

Walker, H. M., Irvin, L., Noell, J., & Singer, G. (1992). A construct score approach to the assessment of social competence: Rationale, technological considerations, and anticipated outcomes. *Behavior Modification, 16*, 448–474.

Walker, H. M., Irvin, L. K., & Sprague, J. R. (1997). Violence prevention and school safety: Issues, problems, approaches, and recommended solutions. *OSSC Bulletin (Oregon School Study Council), 41*(1).

Walker, H. M., Kavanagh, K., Stiller, B., Golly, A., Severson, H.H., & Fiel, E. G. (1998). First Step to Success: An early intervention approach for preventing school antisocial behavior. *Journal of Emotional and Behavioral Disorders, 6*(2), 66–80.

Walker, D. W., & Leister, C. (1994). Recognition of facial affect cues by adolescents with emotional and behavioral disorders. *Behavioral Disorders, 19*, 269–276.

Walker, H. M., & McConnell, S. (1995a). *The Scales of Social Competence and School Adjustment*. Lexington, KY: Thomson Learning.

Walker, H. M., & McConnell, S. (1995b). *The Walker–McConnell Scale of Social Competence and School Adjustment*. Belmont, CA: Wadsworth/Thomson Learning.

Walker, H. M., Nishioka, V., Zeller, R., Severson, H. H., & Feil, E. G. (2000). Causal factors and partial solutions for the persistent under-identification of students having emotional and behavioral disorders in the context of schooling. *Assessment for Effective Intervention, 26*(1), 29–40.

Walker, H. M., Ramsey, E., & Gresham, F. M. (2004). *Antisocial behavior in school: Evidence-based practices*. Belmont, CA: Wadsworth.

Walker, H. M., & Severson, H. H. (1990). *Systematic screening for behavior disorders: User's guide and administration manual*. Longmont, CO: Sopris West.

Walker, H., & Severson, H. H. (2001). *Assessing school engagement and Walker–Severson engagement index*. Eugene: Institute on Violence and Destructive Behavior, University of Oregon.

Walker, H. M., Severson, H. H., & Feil, E. G. (1995). *The early screening project*. Longmont, CO: Sopris West.

Walker, H. M., Sprague, J. R., & Severson, H. H. (2004). School-based violence prevention. In R. H. A. Haslam & P. J. Valletutti (Eds.), *Medical problems in the classroom: The teacher's role in diagnosis and management* (4th ed.). Austin, TX: PRO-ED.

Walker, H. M., Stieber, S., Ramsey, E., & O'Neill, R. E. (1990). Longitudinal prediction of the school achievement, adjustment, and delinquency of antisocial versus at-risk boys. *Remedial and Special Education, 12*(4), 43–51.

Walker, H. M., & Sylwester, R. (1991). Where is school along the path to prison? *Educational Leadership, 49*(1), 14–16.

Wang, M. C., Haertel, G. D., & Walberg, H. J. (1994). What helps students learn? *Educational Leadership, 51*, 74–79.

Wang, M. C., Oates, J., & Weishew, N. (1995). Effective school responses to student diversity in inner-city schools. *Education and Urban Society, 27*, 484–503.

Wasserman, G. A., Keenan, K., Tremblay, R. E., Coie, J. D., Herrenkohl, T. I., Loeber, R., & Petechuk, D. (2003). *Risk and protective factors of child delinquency.* Washington, DC: U.S. Department of Justice, Office of Justice Programs, Office of Juvenile Justice and Delinquency Prevention.

Wasserman, G. A., & Miller, L. (1998). The prevention of serious and violent juvenile offending. In R. Loeber & D. Farrington (Eds.), *Risk factors and successful interventions for serious and violent juvenile offenders.* Newbury Park, CA: Sage.

Waxman, H. C., & Huang, S. L. (1997). Classroom instruction and learning environment differences between effective and ineffective urban elementary schools for African American students. *Urban Education, 32,* 7–44.

Weikart, D. P., Rogers, L., Adcock, C., & McClelland, D. (1971). *The cognitively oriented curriculum: A framework for preschool teachers.* Urbana, IL: University of Illinois.

Wolery, M., Bailey, D., & Sugai, G. (1988). *Effective teaching: Principles and procedures of applied behavior analysis with exceptional children.* Boston: Allyn & Bacon.

Index

"*f*" following a page number indicates a figure or box;
"*t*" following a page number indicates a table